TENTH EDITION

WEST'S PULMONARY PATHOPHYSIOLOGY

THE ESSENTIALS

TENTH EDITION

WEST'S PULMONARY PATHOPHYSIOLOGY

THE ESSENTIALS

John B. West, MD, PhD, DSc

Professor of Medicine and Physiology
School of Medicine
University of California, San Diego
La Jolla, California

Andrew M. Luks, MD

Professor of Medicine
School of Medicine
University of Washington
Seattle, Washington

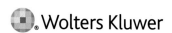

Philadelphia · Baltimore · New York · London
Buenos Aires · Hong Kong · Sydney · Tokyo

Acquisitions Editor: Crystal Taylor
Development Editor: Andrea Vosburgh
Editorial Coordinator: Oliver Raj
Editorial Assistant: Parisa Saranj
Marketing Manager: Phyllis Hitner
Production Project Manager: Bridgett Dougherty
Design Coordinator: Stephen Druding
Manufacturing Coordinator: Margie Orzech
Prepress Vendor: SPi Global

Tenth Edition

Copyright © 2022 Wolters Kluwer.

First Edition, 1977
Second Edition, 1982
Third Edition, 1987
Fourth Edition, 1992
Fifth Edition, 1998
Sixth Edition, 2003
Seventh Edition, 2008
Eighth Edition, 2013
Ninth Edition, 2017

All rights reserved. This book is protected by copyright. No part of this book may be reproduced or transmitted in any form or by any means, including as photocopies or scanned-in or other electronic copies, or utilized by any information storage and retrieval system without written permission from the copyright owner, except for brief quotations embodied in critical articles and reviews. Materials appearing in this book prepared by individuals as part of their official duties as U.S. government employees are not covered by the above-mentioned copyright. To request permission, please contact Wolters Kluwer at Two Commerce Square, 2001 Market Street, Philadelphia, PA 19103, via email at permissions@lww.com, or via our website at shop.lww.com (products and services).

9 8 7 6 5 4 3 2 1

Printed in China

Cataloging-in-Publication Data available on request from the Publisher
ISBN: 978-1-9751-5281-9

This work is provided "as is," and the publisher disclaims any and all warranties, express or implied, including any warranties as to accuracy, comprehensiveness, or currency of the content of this work.

This work is no substitute for individual patient assessment based upon healthcare professionals' examination of each patient and consideration of, among other things, age, weight, gender, current or prior medical conditions, medication history, laboratory data and other factors unique to the patient. The publisher does not provide medical advice or guidance and this work is merely a reference tool. Healthcare professionals, and not the publisher, are solely responsible for the use of this work including all medical judgments and for any resulting diagnosis and treatments.

Given continuous, rapid advances in medical science and health information, independent professional verification of medical diagnoses, indications, appropriate pharmaceutical selections and dosages, and treatment options should be made and healthcare professionals should consult a variety of sources. When prescribing medication, healthcare professionals are advised to consult the product information sheet (the manufacturer's package insert) accompanying each drug to verify, among other things, conditions of use, warnings and side effects and identify any changes in dosage schedule or contraindications, particularly if the medication to be administered is new, infrequently used or has a narrow therapeutic range. To the maximum extent permitted under applicable law, no responsibility is assumed by the publisher for any injury and/or damage to persons or property, as a matter of products liability, negligence law or otherwise, or from any reference to or use by any person of this work.

shop.lww.com

CCS0321

PREFACE

This book is a companion to *West's Respiratory Physiology: The Essentials*, 11th edition (Wolters Kluwer, 2021), and is about the function of the diseased lung as opposed to the normal lung. It was first published over 40 years ago and has therefore served several generations of students. It has been translated into a number of languages.

Building on significant changes from the past edition, including clinical vignettes that emphasizes how the pathophysiology described in the chapter is used in the practice of clinical medicine and expansion of the illustrative material with radiographs, CT images, and color histopathologic sections provided to us by Corinne Fligner, MD, from the University of Washington School of Medicine and Edward Klatt, MD, from Mercer University School of Medicine, this edition includes several new figures and updates to many areas of the book including modern diagnostic and therapeutic approaches. New images have been provided by Sidney Clingerman, BS, and Ann Hubbs, DVM, PhD, from the National Institute of Occupational Safety and Health and the Centers for Disease Control and Prevention; Jeffrey Otjen, MD, from the University of Washington; and Victor Roggli, MD, from Duke University. Data used to revised one of the figures in the book was provided by Marc Houyoux from the United States Environmental Protection Agency. There have also been substantial changes to the multiple choice questions at the end of each chapter. All of the questions in each chapter now adhere to the format used by the USMLE and should be of greater use in preparation for this and similar examinations. The stems of these questions have a clinical orientation, and their purpose is to test the broader understanding of a topic rather than a simple factual recall. Seven 50-minute video lectures related to the material in the book are freely available on YouTube and continue to be very popular (URL: https://meded.ucsd.edu/ifp/jwest/pulm_path/index.html).

As a result of all these changes in the 9th and 10th editions, the length of the book has been increased compared to earlier editions, but its primary purpose has not changed. As before, it serves as an introductory text for medical students in their preclinical and clinical training and remains useful to the increasingly large number of physicians (such as anesthesiologists and cardiologists), advanced practice providers, and other medical personnel (including

v

intensive care nurses and respiratory therapists) who come into contact with patients with various forms of respiratory disease.

As always, we are grateful for any comments on the selection of material or any factual errors and will respond to any e-mails on these subjects.

John B. West, MD, PhD, DSc
jwest@health.ucsd.edu

Andrew M. Luks, MD
aluks@uw.edu

CONTENTS

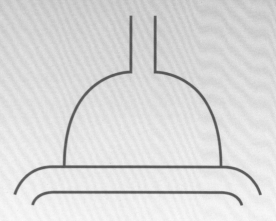

Part 1

Lung Function Tests and What They Mean

We learn how diseased lungs work by doing pulmonary function tests. Accordingly, Part 1 is devoted to a description of the most important tests and their interpretation. It is assumed that the reader is familiar with the basic physiology of the lung as contained in the companion volume, West JB, Luks AM. *West's Respiratory Physiology: The Essentials*, 11th ed. Philadelphia, PA: Wolters Kluwer; 2020.

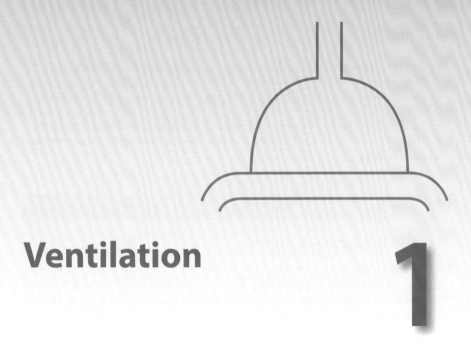

Ventilation

1

The simplest test of lung function is a forced expiration. It is also one of the most informative tests, and it requires minimal equipment and trivial calculations. The majority of patients with lung disease have an abnormal forced expiration volume and, very often, the information obtained from this test is useful in their management. The test has great utility in primary care clinics when patients present for evaluation of chronic dyspnea. For example, it can be valuable in detecting asthma or chronic obstructive pulmonary disease (COPD), extremely common and important conditions. This chapter also discusses a simple test of uneven ventilation. At the end of this chapter, the reader should be able to:

- Describe the utility of the forced expiratory volume in 1 second and the forced vital capacity.

- Distinguish between obstructive and restrictive patterns on the forced expiration maneuver.
- Distinguish between normal and abnormal patterns on the expiratory flow–volume curve.
- Explain the mechanism for effort independent flow at the end of a forced expiration.
- Identify the closing volume and signs of uneven ventilation in a single-breath nitrogen washout test.

TESTS OF VENTILATORY CAPACITY

Forced Expiratory Volume

The forced expiration maneuver, often referred to as spirometry, is the most commonly used test of pulmonary function and yields information used to diagnose disease and monitor progression. The *forced expiratory volume* (FEV_1) is the volume of gas exhaled in *1 second* by a forced expiration from full inspiration. The *vital capacity* is the *total* volume of gas that can be exhaled after a full inspiration.

The simple, classic way of making these measurements is shown in Figure 1.1. The patient is comfortably seated in front of a spirometer having a low resistance. He or she breathes in maximally and then exhales as hard and as far as possible. As the spirometer bell moves up, the kymograph pen moves down, thus indicating the expired volume against time. The water-filled spirometer shown in Figure 1.1 is now seldom used and has been replaced by electronic spirometers, which often provide a graph to be filed with the patient's chart or in their electronic medical record. To perform the test, the patient should loosen tight clothing and the mouthpiece should be at a convenient height. One accepted procedure is to allow two practice maneuvers and then record three test breaths that meet criteria for acceptable results. The highest FEV_1 and FVC from these three breaths are then used. The volumes should be converted to body temperature and pressure (see Appendix A).

Figure 1.2A shows a normal tracing. The volume exhaled in 1 second was 4.0 liters, and the total volume exhaled was 5.0 liters. These two volumes are therefore the forced expiratory volume in 1 second (FEV_1) and the vital capacity (VC), respectively. The VC measured with a forced expiration may be less than that measured with a slower exhalation, so that the term *forced vital capacity* (FVC) is generally used.

These values are reported as both absolute values and as a percentage of what one would predict for an individual of the same age, sex as determined at birth, and height.

The ratio of the FEV_1 to FVC (FEV_1/FVC) is also reported. The normal value is approximately 80% but decreases with age (see Appendix A for normal values). Expert guidelines put forth by various organizations include more refined definitions for the lower limit of normal for the FEV_1/FVC ratio but the 80% cutoff is a useful threshold for the beginning learner.

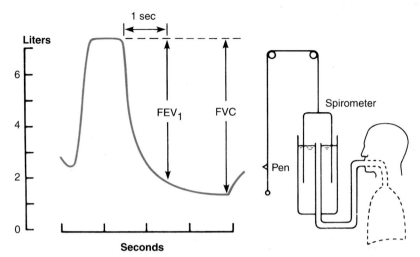

Figure 1.1. Measurement of forced expiratory volume (FEV₁) and vital capacity (FVC).

The FEV can be measured over other times, such as 2 or 3 seconds, but the 1-second value is the most informative. When the subscript is omitted, the time is 1 second.

Figure 1.2B shows the type of tracing obtained from a patient with COPD. Note that the rate at which the air was exhaled was much slower, so that only 1.3 liters were blown out in the first second. In addition, the total volume exhaled was only 3.1 liters and the FEV_1/FVC was reduced to 42%. These figures are typical of an *obstructive* pattern, whereby there is obstruction to airflow, most commonly on exhalation.

The pattern in Figure 1.2B can be contrasted with that of Figure 1.2C, which shows the type of tracing obtained from a patient with pulmonary

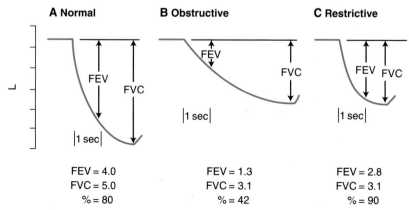

Figure 1.2. **(A)** Normal, **(B)** obstructive, and **(C)** restrictive patterns of a forced expiration.

fibrosis. Here, the VC was reduced to 3.1 liters, but a large percentage (90%) was exhaled in the first second. These figures are consistent with *restrictive* disease, whereby there is some problem limiting, or restricting, the ability of the patient to take an adequately deep inspiration. Note that the specific numerical values in these examples have been inserted for illustrative purposes. These values can vary between patients, but the general pattern will remain the same between patients with each category of diseases.

Forced Expiration Maneuver

- Is simple to perform and yields important data for assessing respiratory function.
- The FEV_1, FVC, and FEV_1/FVC are abnormal in many types of lung disease.
- Can be used to assess the progression of disease or response to treatment.

Bronchodilator Response Testing

If reversible airway obstruction is suspected, the forced expiration test can be performed before and after administering a short acting bronchodilator such as albuterol. In adults, an individual is deemed to have a *bronchodilator response* if either the postbronchodilator FEV_1 or FVC increase by 12% and 200 mL compared to the prebronchodilator values, whereas in children, a bronchodilator response is present if there is a 12% increase in the FEV_1. The presence of a bronchodilator response is helpful in the diagnosis of asthma and in characterizing the physiologic derangements of patients with COPD (see Chapter 4).

Forced Expiratory Flow

This index is calculated from a forced expiration, as shown in Figure 1.3. The middle half (by volume) of the total expiration is marked, and its duration is measured. The $FEF_{25-75\%}$ is the volume in liters divided by the time in seconds.

The correlation between $FEF_{25-75\%}$ and FEV_1 is generally close in patients with obstructive pulmonary disease. The changes in $FEF_{25-75\%}$ are often more striking, but the range of normal values is greater.

Interpretation of Tests of Forced Expiration

In some respects, the lungs and thorax can be regarded as a simple air pump (Figure 1.4). The output of such a pump depends on the stroke volume, the resistance of the airways, and the force applied to the piston. The last factor is relatively unimportant in a forced expiration, as we shall see below.

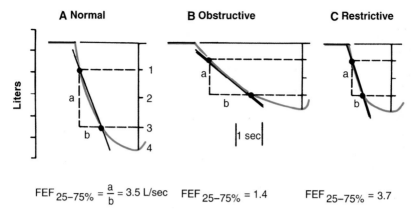

$$FEF_{25-75\%} = \frac{a}{b} = 3.5 \text{ L/sec} \quad FEF_{25-75\%} = 1.4 \qquad FEF_{25-75\%} = 3.7$$

Figure 1.3. A-C. Calculation of forced expiratory flow ($FEF_{25-75\%}$) from a forced expiration.

The *vital capacity* (or forced vital capacity) is a measure of the stroke volume, and any reduction of it affects the ventilatory capacity. Causes of stroke volume reduction include diseases of the thoracic cage, such as kyphoscoliosis, ankylosing spondylitis, and acute injuries such as rib fractures; diseases affecting the nerve supply to the respiratory muscles or the muscles themselves, such as poliomyelitis and muscular dystrophy; abnormalities of the pleural cavity, such as pneumothorax and pleural thickening; disease in the lung itself, such as fibrosis, which reduces its distensibility; space-occupying lesions, such as cysts; or an increased pulmonary blood volume, as in left heart failure.

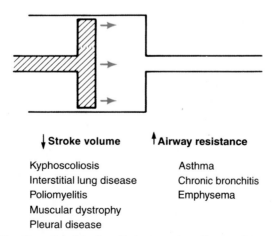

↓ Stroke volume	↑ Airway resistance
Kyphoscoliosis	Asthma
Interstitial lung disease	Chronic bronchitis
Poliomyelitis	Emphysema
Muscular dystrophy	
Pleural disease	

Figure 1.4. Simple model of factors that may reduce the ventilatory capacity. The stroke volume may be reduced by diseases of the chest wall, lung parenchyma, respiratory muscles, and pleura. Airway resistance is increased in asthma and chronic bronchitis.

In addition, there are diseases of the airways that cause them to close prematurely during expiration, thus limiting the volume that can be exhaled. This occurs in asthma and COPD.

The *forced expiratory volume* (and related indices such as the $FEF_{25-75\%}$) is affected by the airway resistance during forced expiration. Any increase in resistance reduces the ventilatory capacity. Causes include bronchoconstriction, as in asthma or following the inhalation of irritants such as cigarette smoke; structural changes in the airways, as in chronic bronchitis; obstructions within the airways, such as a tumor or inhaled foreign body or excess bronchial secretions; and destructive processes in the lung parenchyma, such as emphysema, which interfere with the radial traction that normally holds the airways open.

The simple model of Figure 1.4 introduces the factors limiting the ventilatory capacity of the diseased lung, but we need to refine the model to obtain a better understanding. For example, the airways are actually *inside*, not *outside*, the pump, as shown in Figure 1.4.

Expiratory Flow–Volume Curve

Additional useful information comes from the flow–volume curve. If we record flow rate and volume during a maximal forced expiration, we obtain a pattern like that shown in Figure 1.5A. A curious feature of the flow–volume curve is that it is virtually impossible to get outside it. For example, if we begin by exhaling slowly and then exert maximum effort, the flow rate increases to the envelope but not beyond. Clearly, something very powerful is limiting the maximum flow rate at a given volume. This factor is *dynamic compression of the airways*.

Figure 1.5B shows typical patterns found in obstructive and restrictive lung disease. In obstructive diseases, such as chronic bronchitis and emphysema, the maximal expiration typically begins and ends at abnormally high

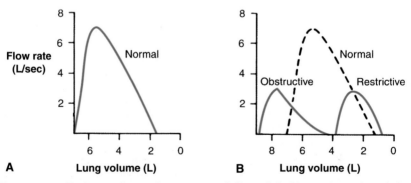

Figure 1.5. Expiratory flow–volume curves. A. Normal. **B.** Obstructive and restrictive patterns.

lung volumes, and the flow rates are much lower than normal. In addition, the curve may have a scooped-out appearance. By contrast, patients with restrictive diseases, such as pulmonary fibrosis, operate at low lung volumes. Their flow envelope is flattened compared with a normal curve, but if flow rate is related to lung volume, the flow is seen to be higher than normal (Figure 1.5B). Note that the figure shows absolute lung volumes, although these cannot be obtained from a forced expiration. They require an additional measurement of residual volume.

To understand these patterns, consider the pressures inside and outside the airways (Figure 1.6) (see *West's Respiratory Physiology: The Essentials*, 11th ed., p. 128). Before inspiration (A), the pressures in the mouth, airways, and alveoli are all atmospheric because there is no flow. Intrapleural pressure is, say, 5 cm H_2O below atmospheric pressure, and we assume that the same pressure exists outside the airways (although this is an oversimplification). Thus, the pressure difference expanding the airways is 5 cm H_2O. At the beginning of inspiration (B), all pressures fall and the pressure difference holding the airways open increases to 6 cm H_2O. At the end of inspiration (C), this pressure is 8 cm H_2O.

Early in a forced expiration (D), both intrapleural and alveolar pressures rise greatly. The pressure at some point in the airways increases, but not as much as alveolar pressure because of the pressure drop caused by flow. Under these circumstances, we have a pressure difference of 11 cm H_2O, which tends to *close* the airways. Airway compression occurs, and now flow is determined by the difference between alveolar pressure and the pressure outside the airways at the collapse point (Starling resistor effect). Note that this pressure

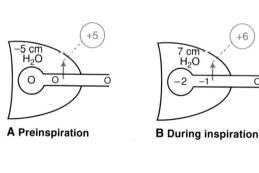

A Preinspiration

B During inspiration

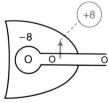

C End-inspiration

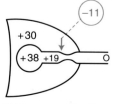

D Forced expiration

Figure 1.6. Diagram to explain dynamic compression of the airways during a forced expiration (see text for details).

difference (8 cm H_2O in D) is the static recoil pressure of the lung, and it depends only on lung volume and compliance. It is *independent* of expiratory effort.

How then can we explain the abnormal patterns in Figure 1.5B? In the patient with chronic bronchitis and emphysema, the low flow rate in relation to lung volume is caused by several factors. There may be thickening of the walls of the airways and excessive secretions in the lumen because of bronchitis; both increase the flow resistance. The number of small airways may be reduced because of destruction of lung tissue. Also, the patient may have a reduced static recoil pressure (even though lung volume is greatly increased) because of breakdown of elastic alveolar walls. Finally, the normal support offered to the airways by the traction of the surrounding parenchyma is probably impaired because of loss of alveolar walls, and the airways therefore collapse more easily than they should. These factors are considered in more detail in Chapter 4.

Dynamic Compression of the Airways

- Limits flow rate during a forced expiration.
- Causes flow to be independent of effort.
- May limit flow during normal expiration in some patients with COPD.
- Is a major factor limiting exercise in COPD.

The patient with interstitial fibrosis has normal (or high) flow rates in relation to lung volume because the lung static recoil pressures are high and the caliber of the airways may be normal (or even increased) at a given lung volume. However, because of the greatly reduced compliance of the lung, volumes are very small, and absolute flow rates are therefore reduced. These changes are further discussed in Chapter 5.

This analysis shows that Figure 1.4 is a considerable oversimplification and that the forced expiratory volume, which seems so straightforward at first, is affected both by the airways and by the lung parenchyma. Thus, the terms "obstructive" and "restrictive" conceal a good deal of pathophysiology.

Partitioning of Flow Resistance from the Flow–Volume Curve

When the airways collapse during a forced expiration, the flow rate is determined by the resistance of the airways up to the point of collapse (Figure 1.7). Beyond this point, the resistance of the airways is immaterial. Collapse occurs at (or near) the point where the pressure inside the airways is equal to the intrapleural pressure (*equal pressure point*). This is believed to be in the vicinity of the lobar bronchi early in a forced expiration. However, as lung volume

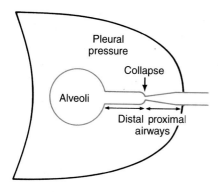

Figure 1.7. Dynamic compression of the airways. When this occurs during a forced expiration, only the resistance of the airways distal to the point of collapse (upstream segment) determines the flow rate. In the last stages of a forced vital capacity test, only the peripheral small airways are distal to the collapsed point and therefore determine the flow.

decreases and the airways narrow, their resistance increases. As a result, pressure is lost more rapidly and the collapse point moves into more distal airways. Thus, late in forced expiration, flow is increasingly determined by the properties of the small distal peripheral airways. In patients with COPD, the collapse point is often in the more distal airways even early in exhalation due to the loss of elastic recoil and radial traction on the airways.

These peripheral airways (say, less than 2 mm in diameter) normally contribute less than 20% of the total airway resistance. Therefore, changes in them are difficult to detect and they constitute a "silent zone." However, it is likely that some of the earliest changes in COPD occur in these small airways, and therefore, maximum flow rate late in a forced expiration is often taken to reflect peripheral airway resistance.

Maximum Flows from the Flow–Volume Curve

Maximum flow ($\dot{V}_{max}$) is frequently measured after 50% ($\dot{V}_{max50\%}$) or 75% ($\dot{V}_{max75\%}$) of the vital capacity has been exhaled. Figure 1.8 shows the abnormal flow pattern typically seen in tests of patients with COPD. The later in expiration that flow is measured, the more the measurement reflects the

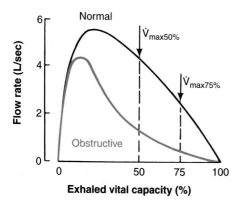

Figure 1.8. Example of an expiratory flow–volume curve in COPD. Note the scooped-out appearance. The *arrows* show the maximum expiratory flow after 50% and 75% of the vital capacity have been exhaled.

resistance of the very small airways. Some studies have shown abnormalities in the $\dot{V}_{max75\%}$ when other indices of a forced expiration, such as the FEV_1 or $FEF_{25–75\%}$, were normal.

Peak Expiratory Flow Rate

Peak expiratory flow rate is the maximum flow rate during a forced expiration starting from total lung capacity. It can be conveniently estimated with an inexpensive, portable peak flow meter. The measurement is not precise, and it depends on the patient's effort. Nevertheless, it is a valuable tool for following disease, especially asthma, and the patient can easily make repeated measurements in the home or workplace and keep a log to show to the their medical provider.

Inspiratory Flow–Volume Curve

The flow–volume curve is also measured during inspiration. This curve is not affected by the dynamic compression of the airways because the pressures during inspiration always expand the bronchi (Figure 1.6). However, the curve is useful in detecting some forms of upper airway obstruction, which flatten the curve because maximal flow is limited (Figure 1.9). Causes include glottic and tracheal stenosis and tracheal narrowing as a result of a compressing neoplasm. In fixed (nonvariable) obstruction, the expiratory flow–volume curve is also flattened.

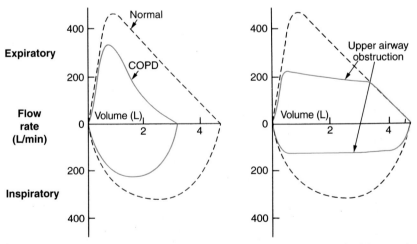

Figure 1.9. Expiratory and inspiratory flow–volume curves. In normal subjects and patients with COPD, inspiratory flow rates are normal (or nearly so). In fixed upper airway obstruction, both inspiratory and expiratory flow rates are reduced.

TESTS OF UNEVEN VENTILATION

Single-Breath Nitrogen Test

The tests described so far measure ventilatory capacity. The single-breath nitrogen test measures inequality of ventilation. This topic is somewhat different but is conveniently described here.

Suppose an individual takes a vital capacity inspiration of oxygen, that is, to total lung capacity, and then exhales slowly as far as they can, that is, to residual volume. If we measure the nitrogen concentration at the mouthpiece with a rapid nitrogen analyzer, we record a pattern as shown in Figure 1.10. Four phases can be recognized. In the first, which is very short, pure oxygen is exhaled from the upper airways and the nitrogen concentration is zero. In the second phase, the nitrogen concentration rises rapidly as the anatomic dead space is washed out by alveolar gas. This phase is also short.

The third phase consists of alveolar gas, and the tracing is nearly flat with a small upward slope in healthy individuals. This portion is often known as the alveolar plateau. In patients with uneven ventilation, the third phase is steeper, and the slope is a measure of the inequality of ventilation. It is expressed as the

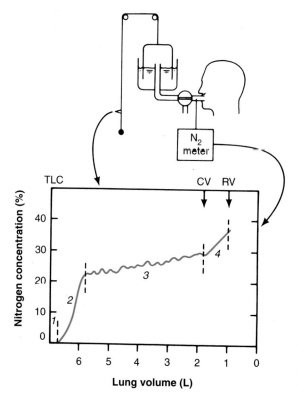

Figure 1.10. Single-breath nitrogen test of uneven ventilation. Note the four phases of the expired tracing. *TLC*, total lung capacity; *CV*, closing volume; *RV*, residual volume.

percentage increase in nitrogen concentration per liter of expired volume. In carrying out this test, the expiratory flow rate should be no more than 0.5 L/sec in order to reduce the variability of the results.

The reason for the rise in nitrogen concentration in phase 4 is that some regions of lung are poorly ventilated and therefore receive relatively little of the breath of oxygen. These areas therefore have a relatively high concentration of nitrogen because there is less oxygen to dilute this gas. Also, these poorly ventilated regions tend to empty last.

Three possible mechanisms of uneven ventilation are shown in Figure 1.11. In A, the region is poorly ventilated because of partial obstruction of its airway, and because of this high resistance, the region empties late. In fact, the rate of emptying of such a region is determined by its time constant, which is given by the product of its airway resistance (R) and compliance (C). The larger the time constant (RC), the longer it takes to empty. This mechanism is known as *parallel* inequality of ventilation.

Figure 1.11B shows the mechanism known as *series* inequality. Here, there is a dilation of peripheral airspaces, which causes differences of ventilation *along* the air passages of a lung unit. In this context, we should recall that inspired gas reaches the terminal bronchioles by convective flow, that is, like water running through a hose, but its subsequent movement to the alveoli is chiefly accomplished by diffusion within the airways. Normally, the distances are so short that nearly complete equilibration of gas concentrations is established quickly. However, if the small airways enlarge, as occurs, for example, in centriacinar emphysema (see Figure 4.4), the concentration of inspired gas in the most distal airways may remain low. Again, these poorly ventilated regions empty last.

Figure 1.11C shows another form of series inequality that occurs when some lung units receive their inspired gas from neighboring units rather than from the large airways. This is known as collateral ventilation and appears to be an important process in COPD and asthma.

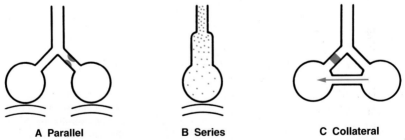

A Parallel   **B Series**   **C Collateral**

Figure 1.11. Three mechanisms of uneven ventilation. In parallel inequality **(A)**, flow to regions with long time constants is reduced. In series inequality **(B)**, dilation of a small airway may result in incomplete diffusion along a terminal lung unit. Collateral ventilation **(C)** may also cause series inequality.

> **Uneven Ventilation**
>
> - Occurs in many patients with lung disease
> - Is an important factor contributing to impaired gas exchange
> - Is conveniently measured with the single-breath N_2 test

There is still uncertainty about the relative importance of parallel and series inequality. It is likely that both operate to a small extent in people with normal ventilation and to a much greater degree in patients with obstructive pulmonary disease. Whatever the mechanism, the single-breath nitrogen test is a simple, rapid, and reliable way of measuring the degree of uneven ventilation in the lung. This is increased in most obstructive and many restrictive types of lung disease (see Chapters 4 and 5).

Closing Volume

Toward the end of the vital capacity expiration shown in Figure 1.10, the nitrogen concentration rises abruptly, signaling the onset of airway closure, or phase 4. The lung volume at which phase 4 begins is called the *closing volume*, and the closing volume plus the residual volume is known as the *closing capacity*. In practice, the onset of phase 4 is obtained by drawing a straight line through the alveolar plateau (phase 3) and noting the last point of departure of the nitrogen tracing from this line.

Unfortunately, the junction between phases 3 and 4 is seldom as clear-cut as in Figure 1.10, and there is considerable variation of this volume when the test is repeated by a patient. The test is most useful in the presence of small amounts of disease because severe disease distorts the tracing so much that the closing volume cannot be identified.

The mechanism of the onset of phase 4 is still uncertain but is believed to be closure of small airways in the lowest part of the lung. At residual volume just before the single breath of oxygen is inhaled, the nitrogen concentration is virtually uniform throughout the lung, but the basal alveoli are much smaller than the apical alveoli in the upright subject because of distortion of the lung by its weight. Indeed, the lowest portions are compressed so much that the small airways in the region of the respiratory bronchioles are closed. However, at the end of a vital capacity inspiration, all the alveoli are approximately the same size. Thus, the nitrogen at the base is diluted much more than that of the apex by the breath of oxygen.

During the subsequent expiration, the upper and lower zones empty together and the expired nitrogen concentration is nearly constant (Figure 1.10). As soon as dependent airways begin to close, however, the higher nitrogen concentration in the upper zones preferentially affects the expired concentration, causing an abrupt rise. Moreover, as airway closure proceeds up the lung, the expired nitrogen progressively increases.

Some studies show that in some subjects, the closing volume is the same in the weightlessness of space as in normal gravity. This finding suggests that compression of a dependent lung is not always the mechanism.

The volume at which airways close is age dependent, being as low as 10% of the vital capacity in young normal subjects but increasing to 40% (i.e., approximately the FRC) at about the age of 65 years. There is some evidence that the test is sensitive to small amounts of disease. For example, apparently healthy cigarette smokers sometimes have increased closing volumes when their ventilatory capacity is normal. Closing volume is often increased in very obese individuals due to premature airway closure at the lung bases.

Other Tests of Uneven Ventilation

Uneven ventilation can also be measured by a multibreath nitrogen washout during oxygen breathing. Topographic inequality of ventilation can be determined using radioactive xenon. This chapter is confined to single-breath tests; other measurements are referred to in Chapter 3.

Tests of Early Airway Disease

Over the years, there has been interest in using some of the tests described in this chapter to identify patients with early airway disease, because once a patient develops the full picture of COPD, considerable, irreversible parenchymal damage has already been done. The hope has been that by identifying disease at an early stage, its progression can be slowed, for example, by cessation of cigarette smoking.

Among the tests that have been examined in this context are the $FEF_{25-75\%}$, and $\dot{V}_{max75\%}$, and the closing volume. Assessment of these tests is difficult because it depends on prospective studies and large control groups. The clinical utility of these tests for identifying early airway disease has yet to be established, and measurement of the FEV_1 and FVC remains the cornerstone of identifying patients with impaired ventilatory capacity.

KEY CONCEPTS

1. The 1-second forced expiratory volume and the forced vital capacity are easy tests to do, require little equipment, and are often very informative.

2. Dynamic compression of the airways causes flow to be independent of effort and is a major source of disability in patients with COPD.

3. The small airways (less than 2 mm in diameter) are often the site of early airway disease, but the changes are difficult to detect.

4. Uneven ventilation is common in airway diseases and can be measured with a single-breath N_2 test.

5. The closing volume is often increased in mild airway disease, and it also increases with age.

CLINICAL VIGNETTE

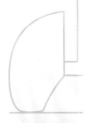

A 30-year-old man complains of increasing dyspnea over a 2-week period. He states that he is no longer able to maintain the same pace on his daily runs and adds that he feels more out of breath when he lies flat on his back at night. He is a nonsmoker and works as a software designer. He also notes that he has been sweating more than usual when he sleeps at night and has lost about 3 kg of weight despite not changing his diet or physical activity. On physical examination, he has no wheezing on auscultation. When he is placed in the supine position for the cardiac examination, he is noted to have increased dyspnea, which resolves when he reassumes the upright position. Spirometry shows the following:

Parameter	Predicted Value	Prebron-chodilator	% Predicted	Postbron-chodilator	% Predicted
FEV₁ (L)	4.5	2.9	64	3.1	69
FVC (L)	5.2	4.2	81	4.2	81
FEV₁/FVC	0.87	0.69	—	74	—

Flow–volume curve:

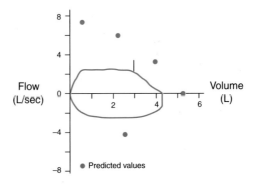

Questions

- How would you interpret the numerical values from his spirometry?
- Are there any changes in his pulmonary function with bronchodilator administration?
- What information does the flow–volume curve add about the cause of his problem?

QUESTIONS

For each question, choose the best answer.

1. A patient performs spirometry as part of an evaluation for a 1-year history of worsening dyspnea on exertion. A graph of expired volume vs. time is shown in the figure below. Data obtained from a healthy individual of the same age, sex, and height are shown on the right for comparison.

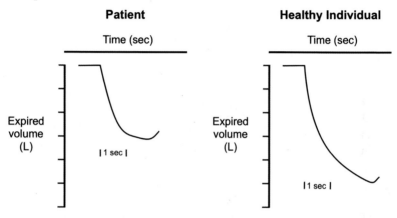

Which of the following diseases would be consistent with the patient's results?
A. Pulmonary fibrosis
B. Asthma
C. Chronic bronchitis
D. Chronic thromboembolic pulmonary hypertension
E. Emphysema

2. A 59-year-old man, who resides at sea level and has a long history of cigarette use, presents for evaluation of chronic dyspnea. On examination, he has an peripheral oxygen saturation (S_pO_2) of 95% breathing ambient air, scattered, polyphonic expiratory wheezes, and a prolonged expiratory phase. Spirometry is obtained in clinic and reveals an FEV_1 1.5 L, FVC 3.1 L, and an FEV_1/FVC 0.48. Which of the following would you expect to find on further pulmonary function testing in this individual?
A. Flattening of the expiratory limb of the flow–volume curve
B. Flattening of phase 3 of the single-breath nitrogen washout
C. Increased closing volume
D. Increased $FEF_{25-75\%}$
E. Increased peak expiratory flow rate

3. A 75-year-old patient performs a single-breath nitrogen washout test as part of evaluation of exercise intolerance. The results are displayed in the figure below. Which of the following best accounts for the observed slope of phase 3 for the patient (*grey line*) in comparison to a healthy control (*black line*)?

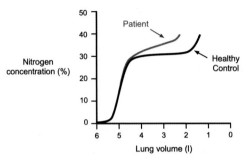

A. Decreased arterial partial pressure of oxygen
B. Decreased hemoglobin concentration
C. Increased airway secretions
D. Increased arterial partial pressure of carbon dioxide
E. Thinning of the airway walls

4. A 72-year-old woman who is a heavy smoker complains of worsening dyspnea and a productive cough over a 9-month period. Spirometry shows an FEV_1 1.1 L, FVC 2.8 L and an FEV_1/FVC 0.39. Which of the following mechanisms best accounts for the results of these tests:
A. Decreased lung compliance
B. Dynamic compression of the airways
C. Increased radial traction on the airways
D. Increased thickness of the blood–gas barrier
E. Weakness of the diaphragm

5. A 61-year-old man with a 30 pack-year history of smoking complains of worsening dyspnea and a dry cough over a 6-month period. Spirometry shows an FEV_1 of 1.9 L, an FVC of 2.2 L, and an FEV_1/FVC ratio of 0.86. Which of the following diseases is consistent with this presentation?
A. Asthma
B. Chronic bronchitis
C. Chronic obstructive pulmonary disease
D. Pulmonary fibrosis
E. Pulmonary hypertension

6. A 41-year-old woman performs spirometry as part of an evaluation for chronic dyspnea. She did not give a full effort on the first test and was asked by the laboratory technologist to repeat the test a second time.

Which of the following changes in her spirometry would you expect to see if she makes a better effort on the second trial?
A. Decreased vital capacity
B. Flattening of the expiratory limb of the flow volume curve
C. Flattening of the inspiratory limb of the flow volume curve
D. Increased expiratory flow at end exhalation
E. Increased peak expiratory flow rate

7. A 57-year-old man undergoes spirometry because of chronic dyspnea on exertion. The flow volume curve is depicted in the figure below. The blue dots show the predicted values. Which of the following factors could account for the shape of the flow–volume curve?

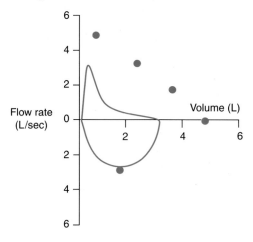

A. Fibrosis of the lung parenchyma
B. Increased radial traction on the airways
C. Increased elastic recoil
D. Increased airway secretions
E. Increased number of pulmonary capillaries

8. A 50-year-old patient, who is a life-long nonsmoker, is undergoing evaluation for chronic hypoventilation and pulmonary hypertension. On chest auscultation, there are no rhonchi or wheezes. A chest radiograph performed as part of the evaluation is shown in the figure below. Panel A shows the original radiograph. Panel B shows the same radiograph with the ribs highlighted by the white lines and the spine outlined by the black line.

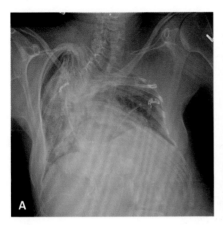
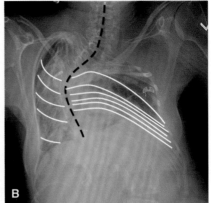

Which of the following would you expect to find on tests of ventilatory capacity in this patient?

A. Decreased $FEF_{25-75\%}$
B. Decreased FVC
C. Decreased FEV_1/FVC
D. Increased closing volume
E. Flattening of the expiratory and inspiratory limbs of the flow volume curve

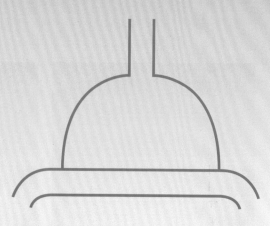

Gas Exchange

2

Chapter 1 dealt with the simplest test of lung function: the forced expiration. In addition, we looked briefly at the single-breath test of uneven ventilation. In this chapter, we turn to the most important measurement in the management of respiratory failure: arterial blood gases. Another test of gas exchange, the diffusing capacity, is also discussed.

At the end of this chapter, the reader should be able to:

- Use clinical and laboratory data to identify the cause of hypoxemia.
- Predict the effect of changes in ventilation on the arterial P$_{CO_2}$.
- Delineate the causes of hypoventilation.
- Describe the effects of ventilation–perfusion mismatch on the arterial P$_{O_2}$ and P$_{CO_2}$.
- Interpret arterial blood gas data to determine the acid–base disturbance.
- Identify causes of reduced diffusing capacity for carbon monoxide.

BLOOD GASES

Arterial P_{O_2}

Measurement
It is often essential to know the partial pressure of oxygen in the arterial blood of acutely ill patients. With modern blood gas electrodes, the measurement of arterial P_{O_2} is relatively simple, and the test is mandatory in the management of patients with respiratory failure.

Arterial blood is usually taken by puncturing the radial artery or from an indwelling radial artery catheter. The P_{O_2} is measured by the polarographic principle, that is, the test measures the current that flows when a small voltage is applied to electrodes.

Normal Values
The normal value for P_{O_2} in young adults residing at sea level averages approximately from 90 to 95 mm Hg, with a range of approximately 85 to 100 mm Hg. The normal value decreases steadily with age, and the average is approximately 85 mm Hg at age 60 years. The fall in P_{O_2} with advancing age is probably due to increasing ventilation–perfusion inequality (see the section later in this chapter). For any given age, lower values are expected at high altitude with the range of normal varying based on the elevation.

Whenever we report an arterial P_{O_2} value, we should have the oxygen dissociation curve at the back of our minds. Figure 2.1 reminds us of two anchor points on the normal curve. One is arterial blood (P_{O_2}, 100 mm Hg; O_2 saturation, 97%) and the other is mixed venous blood (P_{O_2}, 40 mm Hg; O_2 saturation, 75%). Also, we should recall that above 60 mm Hg, the O_2 saturation exceeds 90% and the curve is fairly flat. The curve is shifted to the right by an increase in temperature, P_{CO_2}, and H^+ concentration (these all occur in exercising muscle when enhanced unloading of O_2 is advantageous). The curve is also shifted to the right by an increase in 2,3-diphosphoglycerate (DPG) inside the red cells. 2,3-DPG is depleted in stored blood but is increased in prolonged hypoxia.

Causes of Hypoxemia
There are four primary causes of a reduced P_{O_2} in arterial blood:

1. Hypoventilation
2. Diffusion impairment
3. Shunt
4. Ventilation–perfusion inequality

A fifth cause, reduction of inspired P_{O_2}, is seen only in special circumstances such as at high altitude or when breathing a gas mixture with a low oxygen concentration.

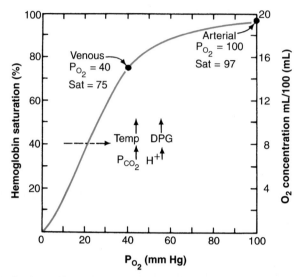

Figure 2.1. Anchor points of the oxygen dissociation curve. The curve is shifted to the right by an increase in temperature, P_{CO_2}, H^+, and 2,3-DPG. The oxygen concentration scale is based on a hemoglobin concentration of 14.5 g/100 mL.

Hypoventilation This refers to a situation in which the volume of fresh gas going to the alveoli per unit time (alveolar ventilation) is reduced. If the resting oxygen consumption is not correspondingly reduced, hypoxemia inevitably results. Hypoventilation is commonly caused by diseases outside the lungs (in which case the lungs are normal) but can also be seen with severe forms of lung disease such as advanced chronic obstructive pulmonary disease (COPD) or pulmonary fibrosis. In addition, hypoventilation is seen in some patients with very high body mass index who have somnolence, polycythemia, and excessive appetite. This has been dubbed the "pickwickian syndrome" after the character, Joe, in Charles Dickens's *Pickwick Papers*. The cause of the hypoventilation is uncertain, but the increased work of breathing associated with obesity is probably a factor, although some patients appear to have an abnormality of the central nervous system. There is also a rare condition of idiopathic hypoventilation known as Ondine's curse. The causes of hypoventilation are shown in Figure 2.2 and listed in Table 2.1.

Two cardinal physiologic features of hypoventilation should be emphasized. First, it *always* causes a rise in P_{CO_2}, and this is a valuable diagnostic feature. The relationship between the arterial P_{CO_2} and the level of alveolar ventilation in the normal lung is a simple one and is given by the *alveolar ventilation equation*:

$$P_{CO_2} = \frac{\dot{V}_{CO_2}}{\dot{V}_A} \cdot K \qquad \text{(Eq. 2.1)}$$

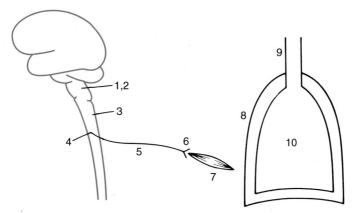

Figure 2.2. Causes of hypoventilation. (See Table 2.1 for details.)

where $\dot{V}_{CO_2}$ is the CO_2 output, $\dot{V}_A$ is the alveolar ventilation, and K is a constant (see Appendix A for a list of symbols). This means that if the alveolar ventilation is halved, the P_{CO_2} is doubled. If the patient does not have a raised arterial P_{CO_2}, he or she is not hypoventilating!

Second, the hypoxemia due to hypoventilation can be abolished easily by increasing the inspired P_{O_2} by delivering oxygen via nasal cannula, face mask, or other devices. This can be seen from the *alveolar gas equation*:

$$P_{A_{O_2}} = P_{I_{O_2}} - \frac{P_{A_{CO_2}}}{R} + F \qquad \text{(Eq. 2.2)}$$

where F is a small correction factor that can be ignored. We will also assume that the alveolar and arterial P_{CO_2} values are the same. This equation states

Table 2.1 Some Causes of Hypoventilation (see Figure 2.3)

1. Depression of the respiratory center by drugs (e.g., barbiturates and opiates)
2. Diseases of the medulla (e.g., encephalitis, hemorrhage, neoplasms [rare])
3. Abnormalities of the spinal cord (e.g., high cervical spinal cord injury)
4. Anterior horn cell disease (e.g., poliomyelitis)
5. Diseases of the nerves to the respiratory muscles (e.g., Guillain-Barré syndrome, amyotrophic lateral sclerosis)
6. Diseases of the myoneural junction (e.g., myasthenia gravis, anticholinesterase poisoning)
7. Diseases of the respiratory muscles (e.g., Duchenne muscular dystrophy, diaphragmatic paralysis)
8. Thoracic cage abnormalities (e.g., severe flail chest, severe kyphoscoliosis, severe obesity[a])
9. Upper-airway obstruction (e.g., tracheal compression by enlarged lymph nodes)
10. Severe parenchymal lung disease (e.g., chronic obstructive pulmonary disease or advanced pulmonary fibrosis)

[a]Some patients with obesity hypoventilation syndrome also have abnormalities in respiratory control (areas 1 and 2).

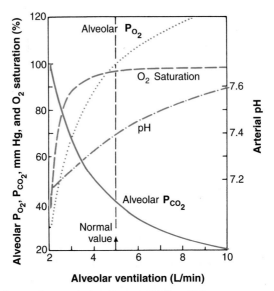

Figure 2.3. Gas exchange during hypoventilation. Values are approximate.

that if the arterial P_{CO_2} ($P_{A_{CO_2}}$) and respiratory exchange ratio (R) remain constant (they will, if the alveolar ventilation and metabolic rate remain unaltered), every mm Hg rise in inspired P_{O_2} (P_{IO_2}) produces a corresponding rise in the alveolar P_{O_2} ($P_{A_{O_2}}$). Because it is easily possible to increase the inspired P_{O_2} by several hundred mm Hg, the hypoxemia of pure hypoventilation is readily abolished. Where possible, the best way to address the hypoxemia due to hypoventilation, however, is to fix the underlying cause of hypoventilation.

It is also important to appreciate that the arterial P_{O_2} cannot fall to very low levels from pure hypoventilation. Referring to Equation 2.2 again, we can see that if $R = 1$, the alveolar P_{O_2} falls 1 mm Hg for every 1 mm Hg rise in P_{CO_2}. This means that severe hypoventilation sufficient to double the P_{CO_2} from 40 to 80 mm Hg only decreases the alveolar P_{O_2} from, say, 100 to 60 mm Hg. If $R = 0.8$, the fall is somewhat greater, say, to 50 mm Hg. Also, the arterial P_{O_2} is usually a few mm Hg lower than the alveolar value. Even so, the arterial O_2 saturation will be near 80% (Figure 2.3). However, this is a severe degree of CO_2 retention that may result in substantial respiratory acidosis, a pH of around 7.2, and altered mental status. Thus, hypoxemia is not the dominant feature of hypoventilation.

Diffusion Impairment

This means that equilibration does not occur between the P_{O_2} in the pulmonary capillary blood and alveolar gas. Figure 2.4 reminds us of the time course for P_{O_2} along a pulmonary capillary. Under normal resting conditions, the capillary blood P_{O_2} almost reaches that of alveolar gas after about one-third of the total contact time of 0.75 seconds available in the capillary. Thus, there is plenty of

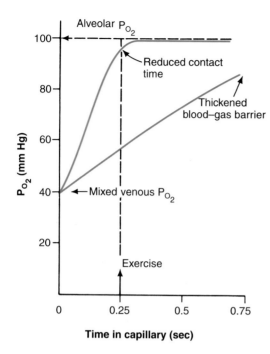

Figure 2.4. Changes in P_{O_2} along the pulmonary capillary. During exercise, the time available for O_2 diffusion across the blood–gas barrier is reduced. A thickened alveolar wall slows the rate of diffusion.

time in reserve. Even with severe exercise, when the contact time may perhaps be reduced to as little as 0.25 seconds, equilibration almost always occurs.

However, in some diseases, the blood–gas barrier is thickened, and diffusion is so slowed that equilibration may be incomplete. Figure 2.5 shows a histologic section of lung from a patient with interstitial fibrosis. Note that the normally delicate alveolar walls are grossly widened. In such a lung, we expect a slower time course, as shown in Figure 2.4. Any hypoxemia that occurred at rest would be exaggerated on exercise because of the reduced contact time between blood and alveolar gas.

Diseases in which diffusion impairment may contribute to the hypoxemia, especially on exercise, include various diffuse parenchymal lung diseases such as asbestosis, sarcoidosis, idiopathic pulmonary fibrosis (cryptogenic fibrosing alveolitis), and nonspecific interstitial pneumonitis, connective tissue diseases affecting the lung including scleroderma, rheumatoid lung, and systemic lupus erythematosus, granulomatosis with polyangiitis (formerly known as Wegener's granulomatosis), Goodpasture's syndrome, and adenocarcinoma in situ. In all these conditions, the diffusion path from alveolar gas to the red blood cells may be increased, at least in some regions of the lung, and the time course for oxygenation may be affected, as shown in Figure 2.4.

However, the contribution of diffusion impairment to the arterial hypoxemia in these patients is less than it was once thought to be. As has been emphasized, the normal lung has lots of diffusion time in reserve. In addition, if we look at Figure 2.5, it is impossible to believe that the normal relationships

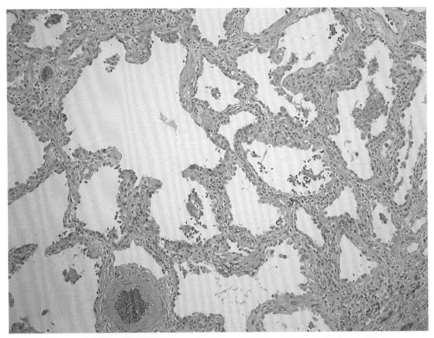

Figure 2.5. **Section of lung from a patient with idiopathic pulmonary fibrosis.**
Note the extreme thickening of the alveolar walls, which constitutes a barrier to diffusion
(compare with Figures 5.1, 5.3, and 10.4). (Image courtesy of Corinne Fligner, MD.)

between ventilation and blood flow can be preserved in a lung with such an
abnormal architecture. We will see shortly that ventilation–perfusion inequality is a powerful cause of hypoxemia, which is undoubtedly occurring in these
patients. Thus, how much additional hypoxemia should be attributed to diffusion impairment is difficult to know. It is clear that at least some of the hypoxemia on exercise is caused by this mechanism (see Figure 5.6).

Hypoxemia could also result from an extreme reduction in contact time.
Suppose that so much blood flow is diverted away from other regions of
the lung (e.g., by a large pulmonary embolus) that the time for oxygenation
within the capillary is reduced to one-tenth normal. Figure 2.4 shows that
hypoxemia would then be inevitable.

Hypoxemia caused by diffusion impairment can be corrected readily by
administering 100% oxygen to the patient. The resultant large increase in
alveolar P_{O_2} of several hundred mm Hg can easily overcome the increased diffusion resistance of the thickened blood–gas barrier. Carbon dioxide elimination is generally unaffected by diffusion abnormalities. Most patients with the
diseases listed earlier do not have carbon dioxide retention. Indeed, typically
the arterial P_{CO_2} is slightly lower than normal because of increases in ventilation mediated by the hypoxemia or by intrapulmonary receptors.

Shunt

A shunt allows some blood to reach the arterial system without passing through ventilated regions of the lung. Intrapulmonary shunts can be caused by arteriovenous malformations such as those seen in hereditary hemorrhagic telangiectasia. In addition, an unventilated but perfused area of lung, for example, a consolidated pneumonic lobule, constitutes a shunt. It might be argued that the latter example is simply one extreme of the spectrum of ventilation–perfusion ratios and is therefore more reasonable to classify hypoxemia caused by this under the heading of ventilation–perfusion inequality. However, shunt causes such a characteristic pattern of gas exchange during 100% oxygen breathing that it is convenient to include unventilated alveoli under this heading. Very large shunts are often seen in the acute respiratory distress syndrome (see Chapter 8). Many shunts are extrapulmonary, including those that occur in congenital heart disease through atrial or ventricular septal defects or a patent ductus arteriosus. In such patients, there must be a rise in right heart pressure to cause a shunt from right to left.

If a patient with a shunt is given pure oxygen to breathe, the arterial P_{O_2} fails to rise to the level seen in healthy subjects. Figure 2.6 shows that although the end-capillary P_{O_2} may be as high as that in alveolar gas, the O_2

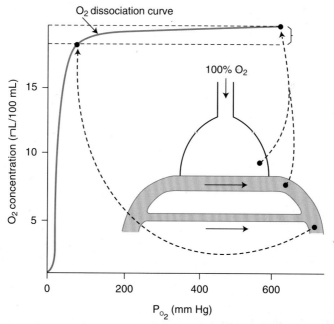

Figure 2.6. Depression of the arterial P_{O_2} by a shunt during 100% O_2 breathing. The addition of a small amount of shunted blood with its low O_2 concentration greatly reduces the P_{O_2} of arterial blood. This is because the O_2 dissociation curve is so flat when the P_{O_2} is high.

concentration of the shunted blood is as low as in venous blood if the shunt is mixed venous blood. When a small amount of shunted blood is added to end-capillary blood, the O_2 concentration is depressed. This causes a large fall in arterial P_{O_2} because the O_2 dissociation curve is so flat in its upper range. As a result, it is possible to detect small shunts by measuring the arterial P_{O_2} during 100% O_2 breathing.

Only shunts behave in this way, and this is a point of practical importance. In the other three causes of hypoxemia (hypoventilation, diffusion impairment, and ventilation–perfusion inequality), the arterial P_{O_2} nearly reaches the normal level seen in healthy individuals during 100% O_2 breathing. This may take a long time in some patients who have poorly ventilated alveoli because the nitrogen takes so long to wash out completely that the P_{O_2} is slow to reach its final level. This is probably the reason why the arterial P_{O_2} of patients with COPD may only rise to 400 to 500 mm Hg after 15 minutes of 100% O_2 breathing.

If the shunt is caused by mixed venous blood, its magnitude during O_2 breathing can be determined from the *shunt equation*:

$$\frac{\dot{Q}_S}{\dot{Q}_T} = \frac{C_{C'} - C_a}{C_{C'} - C_{\bar{V}}} \tag{Eq. 2.3}$$

where $\dot{Q}_S$ and $\dot{Q}_T$ refer to the shunt and total blood flows, and $C_{c'}$, C_a, and $C_{\bar{V}}$ refer to the O_2 concentrations of end-capillary, arterial, and mixed venous blood, respectively. The O_2 concentration of the end-capillary blood is calculated from the alveolar P_{O_2}, assuming complete equilibration between the alveolar gas and the blood. Mixed venous blood is sampled with a catheter in the pulmonary artery. The denominator in Equation 2.3 can also be estimated from the measured oxygen uptake and cardiac output.

Shunt does not usually result in a raised arterial P_{CO_2}. The tendency for this to rise is generally countered by the chemoreceptors, which increase ventilation if the P_{CO_2} increases. Indeed, often the arterial P_{CO_2} is lower than normal because of the additional stimulus to ventilation from hypoxemia.

Ventilation–Perfusion Inequality

In this condition, ventilation and blood flow are mismatched in various regions of the lung, with the result that all gas transfer becomes inefficient. This mechanism of hypoxemia is extremely common; it is responsible for most, if not all, of the hypoxemia in COPD, diffuse parenchymal lung disease, and vascular disorders such as pulmonary embolism and pulmonary arterial hypertension. It is often identified by excluding the other three causes of hypoxemia: hypoventilation, diffusion impairment, and shunt.

All lungs have some ventilation–perfusion inequality. In the normal upright lung, this takes the form of a regional pattern, with the ventilation–perfusion ratio decreasing from apex to base. But if pulmonary disease occurs and progresses, we see a disorganization of this pattern until eventually the normal relationships between ventilation and blood flow are destroyed at the alveolar level. (For a discussion of the physiology of how ventilation–perfusion inequality causes hypoxemia, see the companion volume, *West's Respiratory Physiology: The Essentials*, 11th ed., pp. 76-88.)

Several factors can exaggerate the hypoxemia of ventilation–perfusion inequality. One is concomitant hypoventilation, which may occur, for example, if a patient with severe COPD is overly sedated. Another factor that is frequently overlooked is a reduction in cardiac output. This causes a fall of P_{O_2} in mixed venous blood, which results in a fall of arterial P_{O_2} for the same degree of ventilation–perfusion inequality. This situation may be seen in patients who develop a myocardial infarction with mild pulmonary edema.

How can we assess the severity of ventilation–perfusion inequality from the arterial blood gases? First, the *arterial* P_{O_2} is a useful guide. A patient with an arterial P_{O_2} of 40 mm Hg is likely to have more ventilation–perfusion inequality than a patient with an arterial P_{O_2} of 70 mm Hg. However, we can be misled. For example, suppose that the first patient had reduced ventilation, with the result that the alveolar P_{O_2} had fallen by 30 mm Hg, thus pulling down the arterial P_{O_2}. Under these conditions, the arterial P_{O_2} by itself would be deceptive. For this reason, we often calculate the *alveolar–arterial* P_{O_2} *difference*.

What value should we use for alveolar P_{O_2}? Figure 2.7 reminds us that in a lung with ventilation–perfusion ($\dot{V}_A/\dot{Q}$) inequality, there may be a wide spectrum of values for alveolar P_{O_2} ranging from inspired gas to mixed venous blood. A solution is to calculate an "ideal alveolar P_{O_2}." This is the value that the lung *would* have if there were no ventilation–perfusion inequality and if

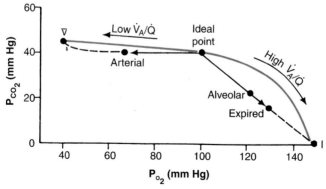

Figure 2.7. O_2–CO_2 **diagram showing the mixed venous ($\bar{v}$), inspired (I), arterial, ideal, alveolar, and expired points.** The curved line indicates the P_{O_2} and P_{CO_2} of all lung units having different ventilation–perfusion ($\dot{V}_A/\dot{Q}$) ratios. (For additional information on this difficult topic, see *West's Respiratory Physiology: The Essentials*, 11th ed., pp. 76-84.)

the respiratory exchange ratio remained the same. It is found from the *alveolar gas equation*:

$$P_{A_{O_2}} = P_{I_{O_2}} - \frac{P_{A_{CO_2}}}{R} + F \qquad (Eq.\ 2.4)$$

using the respiratory exchange ratio R of the whole lung and assuming that arterial and alveolar P_{CO_2} are the same (usually they nearly are). Thus, the alveolar–arterial P_{O_2} difference makes an allowance for the effect of underventilation or overventilation on the arterial P_{O_2} and is a purer measure of ventilation–perfusion inequality. Other indices include the physiologic dead space and physiologic shunt. (See *West's Respiratory Physiology: The Essentials*, 11th ed., pp. 199-202 for further details.)

It is possible to obtain more information about the distribution of ventilation–perfusion ratios in the lung with a technique based on the elimination of injected foreign gases in solution. The details will not be given here, but it is thus possible to derive a virtually continuous distribution of ventilation–perfusion ratios that is consistent with the measured pattern of the elimination of the six gases. Figure 2.8 shows a typical pattern found in young normal volunteers. It can be seen that almost all the ventilation and blood flow go to lung units with ventilation–perfusion ratios near the normal value of 1. As we shall see in Chapters 4, 6 and 8, this pattern is greatly disturbed by various forms of lung disease.

Mixed Causes of Hypoxemia

These frequently occur. For example, a patient who is being mechanically ventilated because of acute respiratory failure after a motor vehicle collision

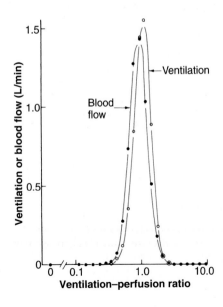

Figure 2.8. Distribution of ventilation–perfusion ratios in a young healthy individual as obtained by the multiple inert gas elimination technique. Note that most of the ventilation and blood flow go to lung units with ventilation–perfusion ratios near 1. (Epublished with permission of the American Society for Clinical Investigation, from Wagner PD, Laravuso RB, Uhl RR, et al. Continuous distributions of ventilation–perfusion ratios in normal subjects breathing air and 100% O2. *J Clin Invest.* 1974;54(1):54-68; permission conveyed through Copyright Clearance Center, Inc.)

may have a large shunt through the unventilated lung (e.g., a large pulmonary contusion) in addition to severe ventilation–perfusion inequality (see Figure 8.4). Again, a patient with interstitial lung disease may have some diffusion impairment, but this is certainly accompanied by ventilation–perfusion inequality and possibly by shunt as well (see Figures 5.6 and 5.7). In our present state of knowledge, it is often impossible to define accurately the mechanism of hypoxemia, especially in the severely ill patient.

Intermittent Hypoxemia

While hypoxemia may last for days to weeks in patients with pneumonia or the acute respiratory distress syndrome or be a permanent problem in some patients with COPD or pulmonary fibrosis, it can also occur in recurrent brief episodes of less than a minute in duration. This intermittent form of hypoxemia is seen most commonly in patients with sleep-disordered breathing, of which there are two primary variants, *central sleep apnea*, where there are no respiratory efforts, and *obstructive sleep apnea*, where, despite activity of the respiratory muscles, there is no airflow.

Central sleep apnea often occurs in patients with severe heart failure and various forms of central nervous system injury and can also be seen in healthy individuals following ascent to high altitude. In one particular form of central sleep apnea, referred to as Cheyne-Stokes breathing, there are alternating periods of breathing, in which the tidal volume waxes and wanes in a crescendo–decrescendo pattern, and periods of apnea. This is thought to occur as a result of instability in the feedback control system that regulates breathing patterns during sleep. The diagnostic hallmark of this pattern on overnight polysomnography is that the periods of apnea are accompanied by absent chest and abdominal wall movements due to cessation of neurologic input to breathing (Figure 2.9).

Obstructive sleep apnea is the more common pattern of sleep-disordered breathing. The first reports were in individuals with very high body mass indices, but it is now recognized that the condition is not confined to them. Airway obstruction can be caused by backward movement of the tongue, collapse of the pharyngeal walls, greatly enlarged tonsils or adenoids, and other anatomic causes of pharyngeal narrowing. With inspiration, the pressure within the airway falls, predisposing to airway collapse. Loud snoring often occurs, and the patient may wake violently after an apneic episode. The diagnostic hallmark of this pattern on overnight polysomnography is that the periods of apnea are accompanied by ongoing chest and abdominal wall movements; despite respiratory effort, air flow ceases due to obstruction of the upper airway (Figure 2.9).

Chronic sleep deprivation sometimes occurs, and the patient may have daytime somnolence, impaired concentration, chronic fatigue, morning headaches, and depression. Untreated patients are at risk for cardiovascular complications such as systemic hypertension, coronary artery disease, and cerebrovascular accidents, possibly as a result of increased sympathetic nervous system activity during apneic episodes and endothelial dysfunction. Application of continuous

Central Sleep Apnea

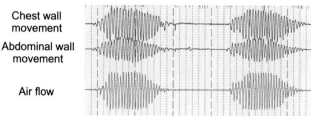

Chest wall
movement

Abdominal wall
movement

Air flow

Obstructive Sleep Apnea

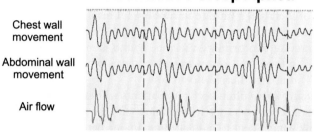

Chest wall
movement

Abdominal wall
movement

Air flow

Figure 2.9. Two patterns of sleep-disordered breathing. The **top panel** shows an example of central sleep apnea. Note that during the period of absent airflow (apnea), there is no movement of the chest wall and abdomen. During periods of breathing, there is often a crescendo–decrescendo pattern to the breathing movements and airflow. The **bottom panel** shows an example of obstructive sleep apnea. Note that during the apneic periods, there is ongoing movement of the chest wall and abdomen.

positive airway pressure (CPAP) by means of a full face or nasal mask during sleep raises the pressure inside the airway, thus acting as a pneumatic splint. While this is generally the most effective treatment, some patients are unable to tolerate it, and surgical approaches may be necessary.

In addition to these pathological forms of intermittent hypoxemia, there has been recent interest in the concept of ischemic preconditioning, whereby brief periods of hypoxemia are intentionally induced as a means of protecting against subsequent ischemic injury as might occur in a myocardial infarction or acute limb ischemia due to peripheral vascular disease.

Oxygen Delivery to Tissues

Although the P_{O_2} of arterial blood is of great importance, other factors enter into the delivery of oxygen to the tissues. For example, a reduced arterial P_{O_2} is clearly more detrimental in a patient with a hemoglobin of 5 g/100 mL than it is in a patient with a normal O_2 capacity. The delivery of oxygen to the tissues depends on the oxygen concentration of the blood, the cardiac output, and the distribution of blood flow to the periphery. These factors are discussed further in Chapter 9.

Arterial P$_{CO_2}$

Measurement

A P$_{CO_2}$ electrode is essentially a glass pH electrode. This is surrounded by a bicarbonate buffer, which is separated from the blood by a thin membrane through which CO_2 diffuses. The CO_2 alters the pH of the buffer, and this is measured by the electrode, which reads out the P$_{CO_2}$ directly.

Normal Values

The normal arterial P$_{CO_2}$ is 37 to 43 mm Hg and is largely unaffected by age. It tends to fall in the late stages of heavy exercise and to rise slightly during sleep. Sometimes, a blood sample obtained by arterial puncture shows a value in the mid-30s. This can be attributed to the acute hyperventilation caused by the pain associated with the procedure and can be recognized by the correspondingly increased pH.

Causes of Increased Arterial P$_{CO_2}$

There are two major causes of CO_2 retention: hypoventilation and ventilation–perfusion inequality.

Hypoventilation

This was dealt with in some detail earlier in the chapter, where we saw that hypoventilation must cause hypoxemia and CO_2 retention, the latter being more important (Figure 2.2). The *alveolar ventilation equation:*

$$P_{A_{CO_2}} = \frac{\dot{V}_{CO_2}}{\dot{V}_A} \cdot K \qquad \text{(Eq. 2.5)}$$

emphasizes the inverse relationship between the ventilation and the alveolar P$_{CO_2}$. In normal lungs, the arterial P$_{CO_2}$ closely follows the alveolar value. Whereas the hypoxemia of hypoventilation can be relieved easily by increasing the inspired P$_{O_2}$, CO_2 retention can only be treated by increasing the ventilation. This may require mechanical assistance as described in Chapter 10.

Ventilation–Perfusion Inequality

Although this condition was considered earlier, its relationship to CO_2 retention warrants a further brief discussion because of frequent confusion in this area. At one time, it was argued that ventilation–perfusion inequality does not interfere with CO_2 elimination because the overventilated regions make up for the underventilated areas. This is a fallacy, and it is important to realize that ventilation–perfusion inequality reduces the efficiency of transfer of all gases, including, for example, the anesthetic gases.

Why then do we frequently see patients with chronic pulmonary disease and undoubted ventilation–perfusion inequality who have a normal or even low arterial P$_{CO_2}$; Figure 2.10 explains this. The normal relationships between

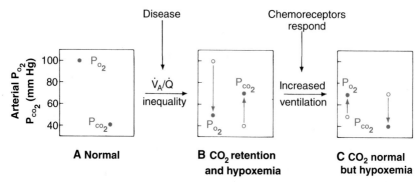

Figure 2.10. Arterial P_{O_2} and P_{CO_2} in different stages of ventilation–perfusion inequality. The normal situation is depicted in panel **A**. Initially, there must be both a fall in P_{O_2} and a rise in P_{CO_2} **(B)**. However, when the ventilation to the alveoli is increased, the P_{CO_2} returns to normal but the P_{O_2} remains abnormally low **(C)**.

ventilation and blood flow (A) are disturbed by disease, and hypoxemia and CO_2 retention develop (B). However, the chemoreceptors respond to the increased arterial P_{CO_2} and raise the ventilation to the alveoli. The result is that the arterial P_{CO_2} is returned to its normal level (C). However, although the arterial P_{O_2} is somewhat raised by the increased ventilation, it does not return all the way to normal. This can be explained by the shape of the O_2 dissociation curve and, in particular, the strongly depressive action on the arterial P_{O_2} of lung units with low ventilation–perfusion ratios. Whereas units with high ventilation–perfusion ratios are effective at eliminating CO_2, they have little advantage over normal units in taking up O_2; despite the high P_{O_2}, oxygen concentration does not increase significantly because hemoglobin is fully saturated with oxygen. The end result is that the arterial P_{CO_2} is effectively lowered to the normal value, but there is relatively little rise in arterial P_{O_2}.

Some patients do not make the transition from stage B to stage C or, having made it, revert to stage B and develop CO_2 retention. What is the reason for this? Generally, these patients have a high work of breathing, often because of a gross increase in airway resistance or increased physiologic dead space. Apparently, they elect to tolerate an increased P_{CO_2}, rather than to expend the extra energy to increase ventilation. It is of interest that if normal individuals are made to breathe through a narrow tube, thus increasing their work of breathing, their alveolar P_{CO_2} often rises.

We do not fully understand why some patients with ventilation–perfusion inequality increase their ventilation and some do not. As we shall see in Chapter 4, many patients with COPD hold their P_{CO_2} at the normal level even when their disease is far advanced. Patients with asthma generally do the same. This can involve a large increase in ventilation to their alveoli. However, other patients allow their P_{CO_2} to rise much earlier in the course of the disease. This likely relates to differences in the central neurogenic control of ventilation and, in particular, the ventilatory response to changes in P_{CO_2} in these two groups of patients.

Arterial pH

Measurement

Arterial pH is usually measured with a glass electrode concurrently with the arterial P_{O_2} and P_{CO_2}. It is related to the P_{CO_2} and bicarbonate concentration through the Henderson-Hasselbalch equation:

$$pH = pK + \log \frac{\left(HCO_3^-\right)}{0.03\, P_{CO_2}} \qquad \text{(Eq. 2.6)}$$

where pK = 6.1, (HCO_3^-) is the plasma bicarbonate concentration in millimoles per liter and the P_{CO_2} is in mm Hg.

Acidosis

Acidemia refers to a decrease in the pH of the blood, whereas the term acidosis refers to a process that leads to decreased pH. Acidosis can be caused by respiratory or metabolic abnormalities or by both (Table 2.2).

Respiratory Acidosis

This is caused by CO_2 retention (i.e., hypercapnia), which increases the denominator in the Henderson-Hasselbalch equation and so depresses the pH. Both mechanisms of CO_2 retention (hypoventilation and ventilation–perfusion ratio inequality) can cause respiratory acidosis. It is important to distinguish between acute and chronic CO_2 retention. A patient with hypoventilation after an overdose of opiates is likely to develop acute respiratory acidosis. There is little change in the bicarbonate concentration (the numerator in the Henderson-Hasselbalch equation), and the pH therefore falls rapidly as the P_{CO_2} rises. The base excess is normal in such cases. Typically, a doubling of the P_{CO_2} from 40 to 80 mm Hg in such a patient reduces the pH from 7.4 to approximately 7.2.

By contrast, a patient who develops chronic CO_2 retention over a period of days to weeks as a result of increasing ventilation–perfusion inequality caused by chronic pulmonary disease typically has a smaller fall in pH. This is because the kidneys retain bicarbonate in response to the increased P_{CO_2} in the renal tubular cells, thus increasing the numerator in the Henderson-Hasselbalch equation. This situation is referred to as a compensated respiratory acidosis. The base excess is increased (greater than 2 mEq/L) in these cases.

These relationships are shown diagrammatically in Figure 2.11. Contrast the steep slope of the line for acute CO_2 retention (A) with the shallow slope of the line for chronic hypercapnia (B). Note also that a patient with acute hypoventilation whose P_{CO_2} is maintained over 2 or 3 days moves toward the chronic line as the kidney conserves bicarbonate (point *A* to point *C*). Conversely, a patient with COPD with long-standing CO_2 retention who develops an acute exacerbation with worsening of ventilation–perfusion relationships may move rapidly from point B to point C, that is, parallel to line A. However, if they are then mechanically ventilated, they may move back to point B, or even beyond.

Metabolic Acidosis

This is caused by a primary fall in the numerator (HCO_3^-) of the Henderson-Hasselbalch equation, an example being diabetic ketoacidosis (Table 2.2). Uncompensated metabolic acidosis would be indicated by a vertical upward movement in Figure 2.11, but in practice, the fall in arterial pH stimulates the peripheral chemoreceptors, thereby increasing the ventilation and lowering the P_{CO_2}. As a result, the pH and P_{CO_2} move along line D.

Lactic acidosis is another form of metabolic acidosis, and this may complicate septic, cardiogenic, or hemorrhagic shock as a consequence of tissue hypoxia. If such a patient is mechanically ventilated, the pH remains below 7.4 when the P_{CO_2} is returned to normal.

Alkalosis

Alkalemia refers to an increase in the pH of the blood, whereas the term alkalosis refers to a process that leads to increased pH. Alkalosis can be caused by respiratory or metabolic abnormalities or by both (Table 2.2).

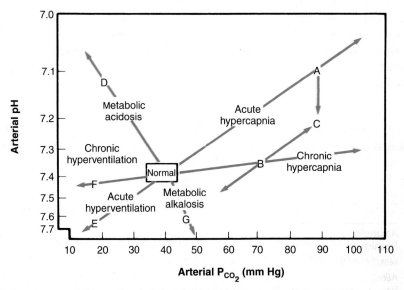

Figure 2.11. Arterial pH–P_{CO_2} relationships in various types of acid–base disturbances. (Modified from Flenley DC. Another nonlogarithmic acid–base diagram? *Lancet* 1971;1:961–965. Copyright © 1971 Elsevier. With permission.)

Table 2.2 Representative Examples of Causes of Primary Acid–Base Abnormalities

Respiratory Acidosis	Respiratory Alkalosis	Metabolic Acidosis	Metabolic Alkalosis

Opiate overdose
Severe chronic
  obstructive
  pulmonary disease
Neuromuscular
  disease
Obesity
  hypoventilation
  syndrome
	Anxiety attack
	High altitude
	Hypoxemic lung
	  disease
		Lactic acidosis
		Diabetic,
		  starvation,
		  or alcoholic
		  ketoacidosis
		Uremia
		Renal tubular
		  acidosis
		Severe diarrhea
			Vomiting
			Loop diuretics
			Excess alkali
			  ingestion
			Hyperaldosteronism

Respiratory Alkalosis

This is seen in acute hyperventilation where the pH rises, as shown by line *E* in Figure 2.11. If the hyperventilation is maintained, for example, at high altitude (Table 2.2), compensated respiratory alkalosis is seen, with a return of the pH toward normal as the kidney excretes bicarbonate, a movement from point *E* to point *F* in Figure 2.11.

Metabolic Alkalosis

This is seen in disorders such as severe prolonged vomiting when the plasma bicarbonate concentration rises, as shown by *G* in Figure 2.10. Usually, there is no respiratory compensation, but sometimes, the P_{CO_2} rises slightly. Metabolic alkalosis also occurs when a patient with long-standing lung disease and compensated respiratory acidosis is ventilated too vigorously, thus bringing the P_{CO_2} rapidly to nearly 40 mm Hg (line *B* to *G*).

Four Types of Acid–Base Disturbance

$$pH = pK + \log \frac{HCO_3^-}{0.03\, P_{CO_2}}$$

	Primary	Compensation
Acidosis		
Respiratory	$P_{CO_2}\uparrow$	$HCO_3^-\uparrow$
Metabolic	$HCO_3^-\downarrow$	$P_{CO_2}\downarrow$
Alkalosis		
Respiratory	$P_{CO_2}\downarrow$	$HCO_3^-\downarrow$
Metabolic	$HCO_3^-\uparrow$	$P_{CO_2}\uparrow$[a]

[a]In some cases, the P_{CO_2} may not increase.

DIFFUSING CAPACITY

So far, this chapter on gas exchange has been devoted to arterial blood gases and their significance. However, this is a convenient place to discuss another common test of gas exchange—the diffusing capacity of the lung for carbon monoxide.

Measurement of Diffusing Capacity

The most popular method of measuring the diffusing capacity (DL_{CO}) is the single-breath method (Figure 2.12). The patient takes a vital capacity breath of 0.3% carbon monoxide (CO) and 10% helium, holds their breath for 10 seconds, and then exhales. The first 750 mL of gas is discarded because of dead space contamination, and the next liter is collected and analyzed. The helium indicates the dilution of the inspired gas with alveolar gas and thus gives the initial alveolar P_{CO}. On the assumption that the CO is lost from alveolar gas in proportion to the P_{CO} during breath-holding, the diffusing capacity is calculated as the volume of $_{CO}$ taken up per minute per mm Hg alveolar P_{CO}.

Causes of Reduced Diffusing Capacity

Carbon monoxide is used to measure diffusing capacity because when it is inhaled in low concentrations, the partial pressure in the pulmonary capillary blood remains extremely low in relation to the alveolar value. As a result, CO

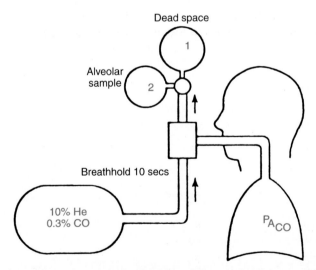

Figure 2.12. Measurement of the diffusing capacity for carbon monoxide by the single-breath method. The subject takes a single breath of 0.3% CO with 10% helium, holds his or her breath for 10 seconds, and then exhales. The first 750 mL is discarded, and then an alveolar sample is collected and analyzed.

is taken up by the blood all along the capillary (contrast the time course of O_2 shown in Figure 2.4). Thus, the uptake of CO is determined by the *diffusion properties* of the blood–gas barrier and the *rate of combination* of CO with blood.

The diffusion properties of the alveolar membrane depend on its thickness and area. Thus, the diffusing capacity is reduced by diseases in which the thickness is increased, including idiopathic pulmonary fibrosis, sarcoidosis, and asbestosis (Figure 2.5). It is also reduced when the surface area of the blood–gas barrier is reduced, for example, by pneumonectomy. The fall in diffusing capacity that occurs in emphysema is partly caused by the loss of alveolar walls and capillaries.

The rate of combination of CO with blood is reduced when the number of red cells in the capillaries is reduced. This occurs in anemia and in diseases that reduce the capillary blood volume, such as pulmonary embolism. It is possible to separate the membrane and blood component of the diffusing capacity by making the measurement at a high and normal alveolar P_{O_2} (see *West's Respiratory Physiology: The Essentials*, 11th ed., pp. 37-40).

Interpretation of Diffusing Capacity

It is clear that the measured diffusing capacity of the lung for CO depends not only on the area and thickness of the blood–gas barrier but also on the volume of blood and concentration of hemoglobin in the pulmonary capillaries. Furthermore, in the diseased lung, the measurement is affected by the distribution of diffusion properties, alveolar volume, and capillary blood. We know that such lungs tend to empty unevenly (see Figure 1.11), so that the liter of expired gas that is analyzed for CO (Figure 2.11) is probably not representative of the whole lung. For these reasons, the term *transfer factor* is sometimes used (particularly in Europe) to emphasize that the measurement does not solely reflect the diffusion properties of the lung. To obtain more specific information about the blood–gas barrier itself in clinical practice, the measured diffusion capacity is adjusted for the hemoglobin concentration and alveolar volume.

Causes of Reduced Diffusing Capacity for Carbon Monoxide

Blood–gas barrier
  Thickened in diffuse parenchymal lung disease.
  Area is reduced in emphysema and pneumonectomy.

Capillary blood
  Volume reduced in pulmonary embolism.
  Capillaries are lost in emphysema.
  Concentration of red cells reduced in anemia.

KEY CONCEPTS

1. The measurement of arterial blood gases (P_{O_2}, P_{CO_2}, pH) is relatively simple with modern equipment and is essential in the treatment of patients with acute and chronic respiratory failure.

2. The four causes of hypoxemia are hypoventilation, diffusion impairment, shunt, and ventilation–perfusion inequality. The last is by far the most common cause.

3. Ventilation–perfusion inequality interferes with the exchange of all gases by the lung including O_2 and CO_2. All patients with this condition have a reduced arterial P_{O_2}, but the P_{CO_2} may be normal or, perhaps, low if ventilation of the alveoli is increased.

4. Acid–base abnormalities include respiratory or metabolic acidosis and respiratory or metabolic alkalosis. These cause characteristic changes in pH, P_{CO_2}, and plasma bicarbonate.

5. The diffusing capacity for carbon monoxide is a useful test of gas transfer by the lung.

CLINICAL VIGNETTE

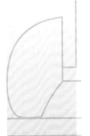

During a period of heavy smoke in the air caused by brush fires in the mountains surrounding her home, a 60-year-old woman with a long smoking history comes to the emergency department complaining of 2 days of increasing dyspnea and cough productive of purulent sputum. She had been seen in the outpatient pulmonary clinic just 2 weeks earlier for regular follow-up of her chronic respiratory issues, and at that time, she had no new complaints and her pulmonary function tests showed the following:

Parameter	Predicted	Prebron-chodilator	% Predicted	Postbron-chodilator	% Change
FVC (liters)	3.9	3.2	82	3.3	3
FEV$_1$ (liters)	3.1	1.3	42	1.4	8
FEV$_1$/FVC	0.79	0.41	51	0.38	48
TLC (liters)	5.8	6.3	109	—	—
RV (liters)	1.9	2.9	152	—	—
DLCO (mL/ min/mm Hg)	33.4	15.7	47	—	—

In the emergency department, her temperature is 37.5°C, heart rate 105, blood pressure 137/83, respiratory rate 24, and S_PO_2

(Continued)

CLINICAL VIGNETTE (*Continued*)

82% while breathing ambient air. On examination, she is talking in short three- to four-word sentences and using accessory muscles of respiration. She has diffuse expiratory wheezes and a prolonged expiratory phase. Her chest is resonant to percussion throughout with limited excursion of the diaphragm on inhalation. Her chest radiograph shows large lung fields, flattened hemidiaphragms, and no focal opacities, effusions, or cardiomegaly. An arterial blood gas is performed prior to placing her on supplemental oxygen and shows the following:

pH	Pa_{CO_2} (mm Hg)	Pa_{O_2} (mm Hg)	HCO_3^- (mEq/L)
7.27	58	50	27

In addition to giving her nebulized bronchodilators and intravenous corticosteroids, she is placed on noninvasive positive pressure ventilation through a tight-fitting mask, after which her dyspnea decreases and she appears more comfortable.

Questions

- How can you relate the abnormalities on spirometry performed in clinic 2 weeks ago to the findings on exam in the emergency department?
- What information does the diffusion capacity for carbon monoxide provide about her lung function?
- How would you interpret her arterial blood gases?
- What is the cause of her hypoxemia at the time of her presentation to the emergency department?
- What change would you expect to see in her arterial P_{CO_2} after she was started on noninvasive ventilation?

QUESTIONS

For each question, choose the one best answer.

1. A 36-year-old man is undergoing evaluation for recurrent epistaxis and gastrointestinal bleeding, a problem from which his father and older brother also suffered. After he was found to have an oxygen saturation of 88% during a clinic visit, he was referred for pulmonary function testing where he had arterial blood gases measured breathing ambient air and an F_IO_2 of 1.0. The results are shown in the table below.

Parameter	F_IO_2 0.21	F_IO_2 1.0
Arterial P_{O_2} (mm Hg)	59	300
Arterial oxygen saturation (%)	88	100

Based on the results of the arterial blood gas analysis, what is the predominant cause of hypoxemia in this patient?
A. Decreased inspired oxygen fraction
B. Diffusion impairment
C. Hypoventilation
D. Shunt
E. Ventilation–perfusion mismatch

2. A 61-year-old woman with chronic obstructive pulmonary disease comes to a hospital at sea level after several days of worsening dyspnea and increasing cough and sputum production. A chest radiograph shows changes consistent with emphysema but no focal opacities. An arterial blood gas is obtained while she is breathing ambient air and reveals: pH 7.41, Pa_{CO_2} 39, Pa_{O_2} 62, and HCO_3^- 23. Which of the following is the cause of her hypoxemia?
A. Diffusion impairment
B. Hypoventilation
C. Low partial pressure of inspired oxygen
D. Ventilation–perfusion inequality
E. Hypoventilation and ventilation perfusion inequality

3. A patient is receiving invasive mechanical ventilation following a drug overdose. After reviewing an arterial blood gas obtained following intubation, the critical care physician changes the tidal volume but leaves the respiratory rate constant. The initial set of parameters is shown in the table below along with the parameters seen after the new settings were initiated. The patient is receiving a medication that causes neuromuscular blockade and cannot take any breaths beyond the set frequency on the ventilator.

Parameter	Initial Settings	New Settings
Tidal volume (V_T, mL)	750	450
Frequency (breaths·min^{-1})	10	10
Dead space volume (V_D, mL)	150	150
Alveolar volume (V_A, mL)	600	300

What percentage of its initial value will the arterial P_{CO_2} be after steady state is reached on the new settings?
A. 33%
B. 50%
C. 100%
D. 150%
E. 200%

4. A 49-year-old man presents to his primary care physician for evaluation of excessive daytime fatigue. He is having trouble staying awake at work during the day and has fallen asleep several times while driving his car. He is accompanied in clinic by his wife who notes that he snores loudly and has intermittent grunts and gasps for air throughout the night. On examination, he has a body mass index of 39 kg/m², a large neck circumference, and crowded oropharynx. He is referred for an overnight polysomnogram, which reveals intermittent periods of absent airflow during which his chest and abdominal wall continue to make respiratory efforts. For which of the following complications is this individual at risk without appropriate treatment?
   A. Anemia
   B. Diabetes mellitus
   C. Emphysema
   D. Hypertension
   E. Pulmonary fibrosis

5. A 63-year-old man, who is a lifelong nonsmoker, presents for evaluation of worsening dyspnea and dry cough over a 1-year period. As part of this evaluation, he undergoes an open lung biopsy. A histopathologic image from this biopsy is shown in the figure below on the left. A comparison from a healthy control is shown on the right.

Patient   **Healthy Control**

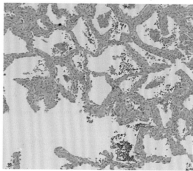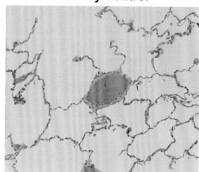

   Based on the histopathologic findings, which of the following would you expect to see on pulmonary function testing in this patient?
   A. Increased closing volume
   B. Decreased diffusing capacity for carbon monoxide
   C. Decreased FEV$_1$/FVC ratio
   D. Increased forced vital capacity
   E. Increased total lung capacity

6. A 56-year-old woman complains of dyspnea on exertion over a several month period. Her pulmonary function tests show an FEV$_1$/FVC ratio of 0.83, total lung capacity 85% predicted, and an uncorrected diffusing capacity for carbon monoxide of 53% predicted. A chest radiograph shows a normal heart size and no focal opacities or effusions. A CT

pulmonary angiogram shows no evidence of pulmonary embolism. Which of the following diagnoses could account for the findings on her evaluation thus far?

A. Asthma
B. Chronic obstructive pulmonary disease
C. Idiopathic pulmonary fibrosis
D. Iron deficiency anemia
E. Sarcoidosis

7. A 48-year-old man is brought into the emergency department with decreased level of consciousness. An arterial blood gas shows pH 7.25, Pa_{CO_2} 25, Pa_{O_2} 62, and HCO_3^- 15. Which of the following could account for the observed abnormalities on his blood gases?

A. Chronic obstructive pulmonary disease exacerbation
B. Diabetic ketoacidosis
C. Gastroenteritis with severe vomiting
D. Morbid obesity
E. Opiate overdose

8. A healthy 21-year-old woman flies from Lima (sea level) to Cuzco, Peru (altitude 3,350 m), on her way to Machu Picchu. Which of the following would likely occur immediately following arrival at Cuzco?

A. Decreased diffusing capacity for carbon monoxide
B. Decreased rate of rise of P_{O_2} in the pulmonary capillary
C. Hypoventilation
D. Increased shunt fraction ($\dot{Q}_S / \dot{Q}_T$)
E. Metabolic alkalosis

9. Which of the following could account for movement from Condition A to Condition B in the figure below:

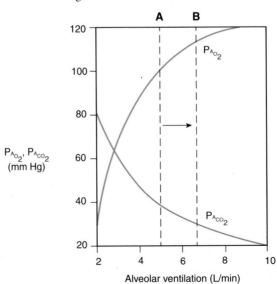

A. Anxiety attack
B. COPD exacerbation
C. Guillain-Barré syndrome
D. Opiate overdose
E. Poliomyelitis

10. At the conclusion of a trek in Nepal, an otherwise healthy 30-year-old woman develops traveler's diarrhea due to an infection with *Campylobacter jejuni*. Two weeks after resolution of her diarrhea and return to home, she develops weakness of her lower extremities, which began in her calves and then extended to her quadriceps muscles. Upon presenting to the emergency department with dyspnea, she is found to have an oxygen saturation of 92% breathing air and a forced vital capacity that is 40% of predicted for her age, sex, and height. Which of the following would you expect to find on further evaluation in this patient?
A. Decreased diffusing capacity for carbon monoxide
B. Decreased serum bicarbonate
C. Increased alveolar P_{O_2}
D. Increased arterial P_{CO_2}
E. Increased pH

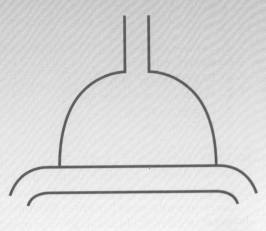

Other Tests

3

In Chapters 1 and 2, we concentrated on two simple but informative tests of pulmonary function: forced expiration and arterial blood gases. In this chapter, we briefly consider some other ways of measuring lung function. Of the large number of possible tests that have been introduced from time to time, we address only the most useful here and emphasize the principles rather than the details of their use. At the end of this chapter, the reader should be able to:

- Predict changes in functional residual capacity, residual volume, and total lung capacity in obstructive and restrictive diseases
- Describe the effect of various disease processes on lung compliance
- Describe the disease processes and other factors that affect airway resistance
- Identify clinical situations associated with reduced ventilatory responses to carbon dioxide and oxygen

- Describe the normal physiological responses to exercise
- Outline the effects of regional differences in ventilation and perfusion on the alveolar P_{O_2} and P_{CO_2}

STATIC LUNG VOLUMES

Measurement

The measurement of the vital capacity with a simple spirometer was described in Chapter 1 (see Figure 1.1). This equipment can also be used to obtain the tidal volume, vital capacity, and expiratory reserve volume (functional residual capacity [FRC] minus the residual volume [RV]). However, FRC, RV, and total lung capacity (TLC) require additional measurements.

These volumes can be measured with a body plethysmograph, which is essentially a large airtight box in which the patient sits. (See *West's Respiratory Physiology: The Essentials*, 11th ed., p. 18-19.) The mouthpiece is obstructed, and the patient is instructed to make a rapid inspiratory effort. As the gas volume in the lungs expands, the air in the plethysmograph is compressed slightly and its pressure rises. By applying Boyle's law, the lung volume can be obtained. Another method is to use the helium dilution technique, in which a spirometer of known volume and helium concentration is connected to the patient in a closed circuit. From the degree of dilution of the helium, the unknown lung volume can be calculated. The RV can be derived from the FRC by subtracting the expiratory reserve volume.

Interpretation

The FRC, RV, and TLC are typically increased in diseases in which there is an increased airway resistance, for example, emphysema, chronic bronchitis, and asthma, although during periods of decreased or absent symptoms, these parameters may be normal in asthma. The RV is raised in these conditions because airway closure occurs at an abnormally high lung volume. Reduced FRC, RV, and TLC are often seen in patients with restrictive disease due to reduced lung compliance, for example, in pulmonary fibrosis. In this case, the lung is stiff and tends to recoil to a smaller resting volume. RV may be normal or even increased when restrictive pathophysiology develops due to diffuse neuromuscular disease.

If the FRC, RV, and TLC are measured by both the plethysmographic and gas dilution methods, a comparison of the two results is often informative. The plethysmographic method measures all the gas in the lung. However, the dilution technique "sees" only those regions of lung that communicate with the mouth. Therefore, regions behind closed airways (e.g., some cysts and blebs) result in a higher value for the plethysmographic than for the dilution procedure. The same disparity is often seen in patients with chronic obstructive pulmonary disease, probably because some areas are so poorly ventilated that they do not equilibrate in the time allowed.

LUNG ELASTICITY

Measurement

The pressure–volume curve of the lung requires knowledge of the pressures both in the airways and in the pleural space (see *West's Respiratory Physiology: The Essentials*, 11th ed., p. 119.) A good estimate of the latter can be obtained from the esophageal pressure. A small balloon at the end of a catheter is passed down through the nose or mouth to the lower esophagus, and the difference between the mouth and esophageal pressures is recorded as the patient exhales in steps of 1 liter from TLC to RV. The resulting pressure–volume curve is not linear (Figure 3.1), so that a single value for its slope (compliance) can be misleading. However, the compliance is sometimes reported for the liter above FRC measured on the descending limb of the pressure–volume curve. The pressure–volume curve is often reported using the percentage of predicted TLC on the vertical axis rather than using the actual lung volume in liters (Figure 3.1). This procedure allows for differences in body size and reduces the variability of the results. Compliance of the entire respiratory

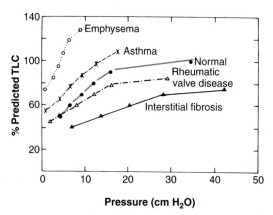

Figure 3.1. Pressure–volume curves of the lung. Note that the curves for emphysema and asthma (during an attack) are shifted upward and to the left, whereas those for rheumatic valve disease and interstitial fibrosis are flattened. (Reprinted from Bates DV, Macklem PT, Christie RV. *Respiratory Function in Disease*. 2nd ed. Philadelphia, PA: WB Saunders, 1971. Copyright © 1971 Elsevier. With permission.)

system is often estimated in patients receiving invasive mechanical ventilation by pausing the ventilator after the desired tidal volume is delivered and measuring airway pressure relative to atmospheric pressure. In such cases, esophageal manometry would be necessary to determine the compliance of the lung parenchyma alone.

Interpretation

Lung elastic recoil is *reduced* in patients with emphysema. Figure 3.1 shows that the pressure–volume curve is displaced to the left and has a steeper slope in this condition as a result of the destruction of the alveolar walls (see also Figures 4.2, 4.3, and 4.5) and the consequent disorganization of elastic tissue. The pressure–volume curve is also typically shifted to the left in patients who are having an asthma attack, but, unlike in emphysema where the change is permanent, the change is reversible in many patients. The reasons for this shift are unclear. Increasing age also tends to reduce elastic recoil.

Some Conditions Affecting Lung Elasticity	
Elastic recoil is *reduced* in	Emphysema
	Some patients with asthma
Elastic recoil is *increased* by	Pulmonary fibrosis
	Interstitial edema

Lung elastic recoil is *increased* in pulmonary fibrosis, which results in the deposition of fibrous tissue in the alveolar walls (see Figures 2.5 and 5.3), thus reducing the lung's distensibility. Elastic recoil also tends to increase in patients with various forms of cardiomyopathy who have a raised pulmonary capillary pressure and some interstitial edema. However, note that measurements of the pressure–volume curve show considerable variability, and the neat results shown in Figure 3.1 are based on mean values from many patients.

AIRWAY RESISTANCE

Measurement

Airway resistance is measured as the pressure difference between the alveoli and the mouth divided by the flow rate. Alveolar pressure can only be measured indirectly: one way to do this is with a body plethysmograph. (See *West's Respiratory Physiology: The Essentials*, 11th ed., p. 205.) The subject sits in an airtight box and pants through a flow meter. The alveolar pressure can be deduced from the pressure changes in the plethysmograph because when the alveolar gas is compressed, the plethysmograph gas volume increases slightly, causing a fall in pressure. This method has the advantage that lung volume can be measured easily almost simultaneously.

Interpretation

Airway resistance is reduced by an increase in lung volume because the expanding parenchyma exerts traction on the airway walls. Thus, any measurement of airway resistance must be related to the lung volume. Note that the small peripheral airways normally contribute little to overall resistance because there are so many arranged in parallel. For this reason, special tests have been devised to try to detect early changes in small airways. These changes include the flow rate during the latter part of the flow–volume curve (see Figure 1.8) and closing volume (see Figure 1.10).

Some Conditions Affecting Airway Resistance	
Resistance is *increased* by	Asthma
	Chronic bronchitis
	Emphysema
	Inhaled irritants (e.g., cigarette smoke)
Resistance is *decreased* by	Increased lung volume

Airway resistance is *increased* in chronic bronchitis and emphysema. In chronic bronchitis, the lumen of a typical airway contains excessive secretions, and the wall is thickened by mucous gland hyperplasia and edema (see Figure 4.6). In emphysema, many of the airways lose the radical traction of the tissue surrounding them because of destruction of the alveolar walls (see Figures 4.1 and 4.2). As a result, their resistance may not increase much during quiet breathing (it may be nearly normal), but with any exertion, dynamic compression (see Figure 1.6) quickly occurs on expiration, and resistance rises strikingly. Such patients often show a reasonably high flow rate early in expiration, but this abruptly drops to low values as flow limitation occurs (see the flow–volume curve in Figure 1.8). Recall that the driving pressure under these conditions is the static recoil pressure of the lung (see Figure 1.6), which is reduced in emphysema (Figure 3.1).

Airway resistance is also increased in patients with asthma. Here, the factors include bronchial smooth muscle contraction and hypertrophy, increased mucous production, and edema of the airway walls (see Figure 4.14). Resistance may be high during attacks, especially in relation to lung volume, which is frequently greatly increased. Airway resistance can be reduced by administration of β2-agonists, which promote bronchial smooth muscle relaxation. Even during periods of remission when the patient is asymptomatic, airway resistance is often raised.

Tracheal obstruction increases airway resistance. This may be caused by compression from outside, for example, an enlarged thyroid or extensive lymphadenopathy, or by intrinsic narrowing caused by scarring or a tumor (fixed obstruction). An important feature is that the obstruction is usually apparent during *inspiration* and can be detected on an inspiratory flow–volume curve (see Figure 1.9). In addition, stridor may be present.

CONTROL OF VENTILATION

Measurement

The ventilatory response to carbon dioxide can be measured with a rebreathing technique. A small bag is filled with a mixture of 6% to 7% CO_2 in oxygen, and the patient rebreathes from this over a period of several minutes. The bag P_{CO_2} increases at the rate of 4 to 6 mm Hg/min because of the CO_2 being produced from the tissues, and thus, the change in ventilation per mm Hg increase in P_{CO_2} can be determined.

The ventilatory response to hypoxemia can be measured in a similar way. In this instance, the bag is filled with 24% O_2, 7% CO_2, and the balance with N_2. During rebreathing, the P_{CO_2} is monitored and held constant by means of a variable bypass and CO_2 absorber. As the oxygen is taken up, the increase in ventilation is related to the P_{O_2} in the bag and lungs.

Both these techniques give information about the overall ventilatory response to CO_2 or O_2, but they do not differentiate between patients who *will not* breathe because of problems with central nervous system control of breathing and those who *cannot* breathe because of mechanical abnormalities of the chest or muscles of respiration. To make this distinction between those who "won't" and those who "can't" breathe, the mechanical work done during inspiration can be measured. To accomplish this, the esophageal pressure is recorded with tidal volume, and the area of the pressure–volume loop is obtained. (See *West's Respiratory Physiology: The Essentials*, 11th ed., pp. 142-143.) Inspiratory work recorded in this way is one useful measure of the neural output of the respiratory center.

Interpretation

The ventilatory response to CO_2 is depressed by sleep, opiate drugs, and genetic factors. An important question is why some patients with chronic pulmonary disease develop CO_2 retention and others do not. In this context, considerable differences of CO_2 response exist among individuals, and it has been suggested that the course of patients with chronic respiratory disease may be related to this factor. Thus, patients who respond strongly to a rise in P_{CO_2} may be more distressed by dyspnea, whereas those who respond weakly may allow their P_{CO_2} to rise and live with a compensated respiratory acidosis. A similar phenomenon of CO_2 retention and depressed ventilatory responses to CO_2 is seen in some individuals with very high body mass indices (BMI).

The factors that affect the ventilatory response to hypoxemia are less clearly understood. However, the response is reduced in many persons who have been hypoxemic since birth, such as those born at high altitude or with cyanotic congenital heart disease. As with CO_2, the ventilatory responses to O_2 are also decreased during sleep, even in healthy individuals.

EXERCISE TESTS

Exercise tests have several important roles. The normal lung has enormous functional reserves at rest. For example, the O_2 uptake and CO_2 output can be increased 10-fold or more when a healthy person exercises, without causing either a fall in arterial P_{O_2} or an increase in arterial P_{CO_2}. Therefore, minor levels dysfunction that may not be apparent at rest may manifest under the stress of exercise. Another reason for exercise testing is to assess disability. Patients vary considerably in their own assessment of the amount of activity they can do, and an objective measurement on a treadmill, stationary bicycle, or a walk along a hallway can be revealing. Exercise tests can help evaluate the primary system limiting exercise when simpler tests such as spirometry or echocardiography do not reveal a clear etiology or when a patient has two significant problems such as COPD and heart disease and it is unclear which is the main source of his or her dyspnea. Finally, specific exercise protocols are also used in the diagnostic algorithms for asthma and coronary artery disease.

Measurement

A commonly performed test is the cardiopulmonary exercise test (CPET) in which the individual exercises on a cycle ergometer or treadmill at steadily increasing levels of work until they reach their maximum exercise capacity. Variables that are measured during CPET include work load, total ventilation, respiratory frequency, tidal volume, heart rate, electrocardiography, blood pressure, O_2 consumption, CO_2 output, respiratory exchange ratio, lactate, and the arterial and end-tidal P_{O_2} and P_{CO_2}. More specialized measurements, such as diffusing capacity and cardiac output, are sometimes made. The physiologic dead space can be estimated from the blood gas and ventilation data using Bohr's method. (See *West's Respiratory Physiology: The Essentials*, 11th ed., pp. 24 and 215.)

The respiratory exchange ratio (R) is not measured directly and, instead, is calculated on a continuous basis from the O_2 consumption and

CO_2 output using current breath-by-breath exercise systems. R is typically about 0.8 in early to mid-exercise but rises above 1.0 when the patient passes his or her *anaerobic threshold* or *ventilatory threshold*. This occurs due to an increase in the CO_2 production secondary to the liberation of lactic acid from the hypoxic muscles. The hydrogen ions react with bicarbonate and lead to an increase in CO_2 excretion above that produced by aerobic metabolism. The fall in pH provides an additional stimulus to breathing.

Submaximal exercise tests (so-called field exercise tests) provide less data than a formal CPET but can also be informative. One is the 6-minute walk test (6MWT), in which the individual is asked to walk as far as possible along a corridor or other flat terrain for 6 minutes. The result is expressed in meters covered and has the advantage that the test simulates real-life conditions. The results often improve with practice. Other field tests include the incremental shuttle walk test, in which the patient walks around two cones placed 10 m apart at a steadily increasing speed set by beeps from an audiotape device, and the endurance shuttle walk test, in which the individual walks as long as tolerated at a constant preset pace. These field tests are only of utility in individuals with limited exercise capacity and are not useful for assessing exercise responses in fit individuals. These tests cannot be used to identify the cause of exercise limitation and, instead, can only be used to monitor response to treatment of degree of limitation over time.

Interpretation

In healthy individuals, the variables noted above demonstrate a characteristic pattern of response with progressive exercise (Figure 3.2). This is often referred to as a "cardiac pattern" of limitation, which refers to the fact that an individual stops exercising because the heart reaches the limit of its ability to deliver oxygenated blood to the exercising muscles before the ventilatory pump reaches its limit. These individuals demonstrate a clear anaerobic or "ventilatory" threshold with a lactic acidosis, and the arterial P_{O_2} remains constant through exercise. The heart rate rises close to the predicted maximum, while the minute ventilation at peak exercise is well below the predicted maximum (maximum voluntary ventilation).

Depending on the disease process and the system limiting exercise, the pattern of responses seen with progressive exercise will vary from that seen in Figure 3.2 (Table 3.1). Patients with different forms of cardiac disease show a similar pattern to that seen in healthy individuals, but the maximum exercise capacity ($\dot{V}o_{2\,max}$) is reduced. Patients with chronic obstructive pulmonary disease cease exercise because the ventilatory pump fails before the heart reaches the limit of its capacity. In addition to not reaching the anaerobic threshold and developing hypoxemia, they demonstrate a rising P_{CO_2} at end exercise, the

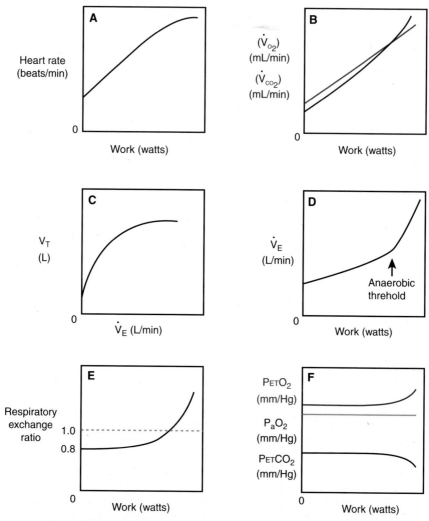

Figure 3.2. Physiological responses to progressive exercise in healthy individuals.
A. Heart rate. **B.** O_2 consumption ($\dot{V}o_2$) and CO_2 output ($\dot{V}co_2$). **C.** Tidal volume (V_T). **D.**
Minute ventilation ($\dot{V}_E$). **E.** Respiratory exchange ratio (R). **F.** End-tidal (ET) and arterial
partial pressures of oxygen and carbon dioxide. End-tidal values are a surrogate measure
of the alveolar partial pressure. With the exception of panel **C**, all graphs show how the
parameter changes as the work rate increases.

hallmark of ventilatory failure. Patients with diffuse parenchymal lung disease
often resemble those with cardiac limitation except they develop hypoxemia
with progressive exercise and can have altered ventilatory responses. Devia-
tions from these basic patterns can be seen depending on the particular disease process.

Table 3.1 Patterns of Exercise Limitation

Parameter	Cardiac Limitation (Healthy)	Cardiac Limitation (Cardiac Disease)	Ventilatory Limitation
$\dot{V}o_{2max}$	Normal	Decreased	Decreased
Heart rate at peak exercise	>80% of predicted maximum	>80% of predicted maximum	<80% of predicted maximum
$\dot{V}_E$ at peak exercise	<80% of predicted maximum	<80% of predicted maximum	>80% of predicted maximum
Attain anaerobic threshold	Yes	Yes	No
Lactic acidosis	Yes	Yes	No
Arterial P_{O_2}	Stable through exercise	Stable through exercise	Decreases
Arterial P_{CO_2}	Decreases at end exercise	Decreases at end exercise	Increases at end exercise

DYSPNEA

Dyspnea refers to the sensation of difficulty with breathing and should be distinguished from simple tachypnea (rapid breathing) or hyperpnea (increased ventilation). Because dyspnea is a subjective phenomenon, it is difficult to measure, and the factors responsible for it are poorly understood. Broadly speaking, dyspnea occurs when the *demand for ventilation* is out of proportion to the patient's *ability to respond* to that demand. As a result, breathing becomes difficult, uncomfortable, or labored.

An *increased demand for ventilation* is often caused by changes in the blood gases and the pH. High ventilations on exercise are common in individuals with inefficient pulmonary gas exchange, especially those with large physiologic dead spaces, who tend to develop CO_2 retention and acidosis unless they achieve high minute ventilation. Another important factor is stimulation of intrapulmonary receptors. This factor presumably explains the high exercise ventilations in many individuals with interstitial lung disease, possibly as a result of stimulation of the juxtacapillary (J) receptors.

A *reduced ability to respond* to the ventilatory needs is generally caused by abnormal mechanics of the lung or chest wall. Frequently, increased airway resistance is the problem, as in asthma, but other causes include a stiff chest wall, as in kyphoscoliosis, or neuromuscular impairment.

The assessment of dyspnea is difficult, largely because it is something that only the individual feels and cannot be measured objectively. A variety of tools are used in both research studies and clinical practice for this purpose. The simplest tool is the visual analog scale in which the individual is asked to place a mark on a horizontal line 100 mm in length indicating the severity of their symptoms. Other scoring systems include the Borg Dyspnea Scale, the Medical Research Council (MRC) scale, the Baseline Dyspnea Index (BDI), and standardized approaches that ask the individual questions such as the type of activities that leave them out of breath, how far they can walk, and whether or not they can keep up with people of the same age. Given the subjective nature of the symptom, comparison of scores between individuals is difficult, whereas following changes in scores in a given individual over time or in response to treatment is more feasible.

TOPOGRAPHIC DIFFERENCES OF LUNG FUNCTION

Measurement

The regional distribution of blood flow and ventilation in the lung can be measured with radioactive substances. (See *West's Respiratory Physiology: The Essentials*, 11th ed., p. 25, 53.) One method of detecting areas of absent blood flow is by injecting albumin aggregates labeled with radioactive technetium. An image of the radioactivity is then made with a gamma camera, and "cold" areas containing no activity are readily apparent. The distribution of blood flow can also be obtained from an intravenous injection of radioactive xenon or other gas dissolved in saline. When the gas reaches the pulmonary capillaries, it is evolved into the alveolar gas, and the radiation can be detected by a gamma camera. This method has the advantage of giving blood flow per unit volume of lung. Special chest CT protocols and MRI scanning techniques can also be used to assess regional variation in blood flow.

The distribution of ventilation can be measured in a similar way, except that the gas is inhaled into the alveoli from a spirometer. Either a single inspiration or a wash-in over a series of breaths can be recorded. This method of assessing ventilation can be combined with the technetium-labeled albumin technique described above to diagnose pulmonary embolism, although this approach has since been supplanted by CT pulmonary angiography as the diagnostic method of choice.

Interpretation

The distribution of blood flow in the upright lung is uneven, being much greater at the base than at the apex (Figure 3.3). The differences are caused by gravity and can be explained by the relationships between the pulmonary arterial, venous, and alveolar pressures. (See *West's Respiratory Physiology: The Essentials*, 11th ed., p. 54.) Exercise results in a more uniform distribution because of the increase in pulmonary arterial pressure; the same result is found in disease conditions such as pulmonary arterial hypertension and

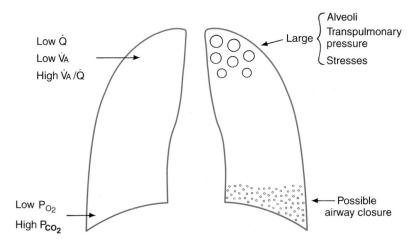

Figure 3.3. Regional differences of structure and function in the upright lung.

left-to-right cardiac shunts. Localized lung disease, for example, a bleb or a bulla, or area of fibrosis, frequently decreases the regional blood flow.

The distribution of ventilation is also gravity-dependent, such that the ventilation to the base normally exceeds that to the apex. The explanation is the distortion that the lung suffers because of gravity and the larger transpulmonary pressure at the apex compared with the base. (See *West's Respiratory Physiology: The Essentials*, 11th ed., p. 118.) Localized lung disease, for example, a bulla, usually reduces the ventilation in that area. In generalized lung diseases—such as asthma, chronic bronchitis, emphysema, and pulmonary fibrosis—areas of reduced ventilation and blood flow can frequently be detected.

Healthy people show a reversal of the normal pattern of ventilation if they inhale a small amount of radioactive gas from RV. The reason is that the airways at the base of the lung are closed under these conditions because intrapleural pressure actually rises above airway pressure. The same pattern may occur at FRC in older subjects because the lower zone airways close at an abnormally high lung volume. Similar findings may be seen in individuals with emphysema, interstitial edema, and obesity. All of these conditions exaggerate airway closure at the base of the lung.

Other regional differences of structure and function also occur. The gravity-induced distortion of the upright lung causes the alveoli at the apex to be larger than those at the base. These larger alveoli are also associated with greater mechanical stresses that may play a role in the development of some diseases, such as centriacinar emphysema (see Figure 4.5A) and spontaneous pneumothorax.

The regional differences in ventilation and perfusion lead to regional differences in the average ventilation–perfusion ratios and, as a result, variation in the average alveolar P_{O_2} and P_{CO_2} (Figure 3.3).

THE ROLE OF PULMONARY FUNCTION TESTS

Some of the tests described in the first three chapters of this book, such as the forced expiration maneuver, lung volume measurements, and CPET, are used quite commonly in clinical practice, while others are used much less often. Regardless of the frequency of use, it is important to remember that these tests rarely lead to a specific diagnosis. Instead, they provide information about the primary physiologic issues in a patient that must be considered along with information obtained from the clinical history, physical examination, chest imaging, and laboratory tests to arrive at a particular diagnosis.

Beyond their role in diagnosis, pulmonary function tests are also valuable for monitoring the progress of a patient, as might occur following lung or hematopoietic stem cell transplantation or after initiation of therapy for a particular pulmonary disease. They are also useful in assessing patients prior to surgical resection of portions of the lung, determining disability for purposes of workers' compensation, and estimating the prevalence of disease in a community or workplace, such as in a coal mine or an asbestos factory.

Whether to perform particular tests depends largely on the clinical problem, their ease and expense, and the likelihood that they will give useful information that either aids in diagnosis or affects patient management in some other way. Tests such as spirometry and arterial blood gases are inexpensive and yield a lot of useful information and, therefore, are used widely in clinical practice, while other tests, such as assessment of lung compliance with esophageal manometry, are more challenging to do and, therefore, are performed with far less frequency.

KEY CONCEPTS

1. Lung elastic recoil is reduced in emphysema and some patients with asthma. It is increased in interstitial fibrosis and slightly in interstitial edema.

2. Airway resistance is increased in chronic bronchitis, emphysema, and asthma. It is reduced by increasing lung volume. Tracheal obstruction increases both inspiratory and expiratory resistance.

3. The control of ventilation by increased P_{CO_2} and reduced P_{O_2} varies greatly among people and may affect the clinical pattern of patients with severe COPD and morbid obesity.

4. The lung at rest has enormous reserves of function, and valuable information can therefore often be obtained during exercise that stresses gas exchange.

5. Dyspnea is a common, important symptom in many lung diseases but can be truly assessed only by the patient.

CLINICAL VIGNETTE

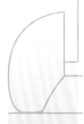

A 30-year-old woman is referred to the pulmonary clinic for evaluation of 6 months of worsening dyspnea on exertion and a nonproductive cough. She had not had fevers, weight loss, or chest pain but had to stop her weekly dance classes due to dyspnea. She is a life-long nonsmoker and has several pets at home including a dog, a cat, and a cockatiel that she received 1 year ago from a friend who had to give it up due to a respiratory disorder. In the clinic, she is afebrile and has a normal heart rate, blood pressure, respiratory rate, and an S_pO_2 of 96% breathing ambient air. The only noteworthy finding on her exam is the presence of fine end-inspiratory crackles in the bilateral lower lung zones. A plain chest radiograph shows faint bilateral opacities, while a follow-up chest CT scan shows diffuse "ground glass opacities" consistent with an alveolar-filling process. Pulmonary function tests show the following:

Parameter	Predi-cted	Prebron-chodilator	% Predicted	Postbron-chodilator	% Change
FVC (liters)	4.37	1.73	40	1.79	4
FEV$_1$ (liters)	3.65	1.57	43	1.58	0
FEV$_1$/FVC	0.84	0.91	108	0.88	−3
TLC (liters)	6.12	2.68	44	—	—
DLCO (mL/min/mm Hg)	15.13	32.19	47	—	—

Questions

- What changes would you expect to see in her FRC and RV?
- If you were able to obtain estimates of pleural pressure using a catheter inserted through her nose into her esophagus, what changes would you expect to see in the pressure–volume curve for her lungs?
- How will her airway resistance compare to that of a healthy individual?
- What would you expect to happen to her arterial P_{O_2} during a cardiopulmonary exercise test?

QUESTIONS

For each question, choose the one best answer.

1. As part of a research project, esophageal manometry is performed to estimate pleural pressure in a patient with a chronic respiratory disease. The difference in pressure between the mouth and the lower esophagus is recorded as the patient exhales in 1-liter increments from total lung capacity. The pressure volume curve for the patient is displayed in the figure below compared to the data obtained from a healthy individual.

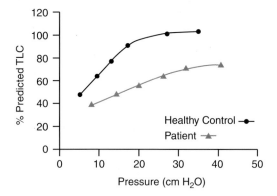

Based on these results, from which of the following chronic respiratory diseases is this patient likely suffering?
A. Asthma
B. Chronic bronchitis
C. Emphysema
D. Pulmonary arterial hypertension
E. Pulmonary fibrosis

2. A 41-year-old woman complains of acute dyspnea and chest pain. She is sent for a ventilation–perfusion scan in which she inhales radiolabeled xenon and receives an injection of technetium-labeled macroaggregated albumin. Using a gamma camera, images are recorded that reflect the ventilation and perfusion throughout each lung. The lung images reveal a homogenous pattern of activity throughout the entirety of both lungs, while the perfusion images show a large area with no activity in the left lower lobe. Based on these results, what is the most likely cause of her dyspnea and chest pain?
A. Asthma exacerbation
B. Chronic obstructive pulmonary disease exacerbation
C. Myocardial infarction
D. Pneumothorax
E. Pulmonary embolism

3. The figure below depicts the changes in lung volume during a forced expiration maneuver.

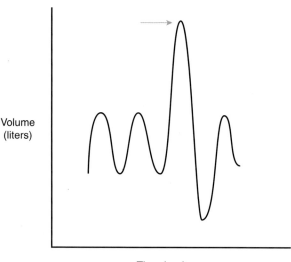

Which of the following parameters reaches its minimum value at the point denoted by the arrow in the figure?
A. Airway resistance
B. Arterial pH
C. Lung elastic recoil
D. Pulmonary vascular resistance
E. Transpulmonary pressure

4. A 65-year-old man with a long history of smoking presents with 1 year of worsening dyspnea on exertion. On auscultation, he has scattered expiratory musical sounds and a prolonged expiratory phase. A chest radiograph reveals large lung volumes, flattened diaphragms, and decreased lung markings in the apical regions, while spirometry shows a reduced FEV_1 and FVC and FEV_1/FVC of 0.62. Which of the following would you expect to observe on further pulmonary function testing?
A. Decreased total lung capacity
B. Decreased airway resistance
C. Decreased lung compliance
D. Increased diffusion capacity for carbon monoxide
E. Increased functional residual capacity

5. A 35-year-old woman undergoes a cardiopulmonary exercise test as part of an evaluation for dyspnea on exertion. Data from the test are displayed in the table below.

Parameter	Rest	End Exercise
Arterial P_{CO_2} (mm Hg)	40	33
Arterial P_{O_2} (mm Hg)	90	65
Heart rate	75	180
R	0.8	1.2
$\dot{V}_E$ (L/min)	8	95

Which of the parameters shown in the table demonstrates a different pattern of response than would be expected in a healthy individual?
A. Arterial P_{CO_2}
B. Arterial P_{O_2}
C. Heart rate
D. Respiratory exchange ratio (R)
E. Minute ventilation ($\dot{V}_E$)

6. A 68-year-old woman undergoes pulmonary function testing as part of an evaluation for dyspnea and chronic cough. When lung volume measurements are obtained using both body plethysmography and helium dilution, the residual volume is found to be 0.6 liters higher when measured by plethysmography than when measured by helium dilution. Which of the following underlying diseases could account for this observation?
A. Asbestosis
B. Chronic obstructive pulmonary disease
C. Heart failure
D. Idiopathic pulmonary fibrosis
E. Neuromuscular disease

7. A 56-year-old man with a body mass index of 42 kg/m² is seen in clinic for evaluation of fatigue and exercise intolerance. He is a life-long nonsmoker. On exam, he has no crackles or wheezes. A chest radiograph shows low lung volumes but no lung opacities. On a forced expiration maneuver, his FEV_1 is 75% predicted, FVC 79% predicted, and FEV_1/FVC 0.82. An arterial blood gas is performed while breathing ambient air and reveals the following:

pH	P_{aCO_2} (mm Hg)	P_{aO_2} (mm Hg)	HCO_3^- (mEq/L)
7.36	55	64	31

Which of the following would you most likely find on further evaluation of pulmonary function in this patient?
A. Decreased closing volume
B. Decreased residual volume
C. Decreased ventilatory response to carbon dioxide
D. Increased compliance of the lung parenchyma
E. Increased ventilatory response to hypoxemia

8. In the figure below, which of the following would you expect to see at the location denoted by the letter A when compared to the location denoted by the letter B?

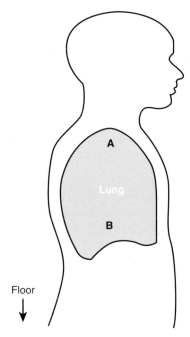

A. Decreased alveolar P_{O_2}
B. Decreased ventilation
C. Decreased ventilation–perfusion ratio
D. Increased alveolar P_{CO_2}
E. Increased perfusion

9. A 71-year-old man is referred for a cardiopulmonary exercise test for evaluation of dyspnea on exertion. His maximum predicted heart rate is 150 beats per minute, while pulmonary function testing performed prior to the exercise test demonstrated that his maximum predicted minute ventilation was 52 L/min. Data from his test are displayed in the table below.

Parameter	Rest	End Exercise
Arterial P_{CO_2} (mm Hg)	40	47
Arterial P_{O_2} (mm Hg)	85	62
Heart rate	75	110
Lactate (mmol/L)	1.6	1.8
R	0.8	0.9
$\dot{V}_E$ (L/min)	8	50

Electrocardiography performed during the test did not show any ST segment changes. Based on these results, which of the following is the most likely cause of his exercise limitation?
A. Chronic obstructive pulmonary disease
B. Ischemic cardiomyopathy
C. Pulmonary arterial hypertension
D. Valvular heart disease

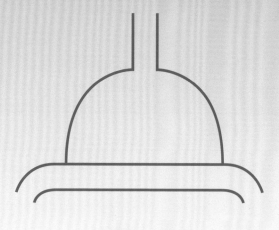

Part 2

Function of the Diseased Lung

This part is devoted to the patterns of abnormal function in some common types of lung disease.

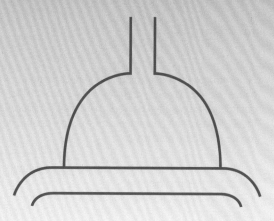

Obstructive Diseases

4

Obstructive diseases of the lung are extremely common and remain an important cause of morbidity and mortality. While the distinctions among the various types of obstructive disease are blurred, giving rise to difficulties in definition and diagnosis, all of these diseases are characterized by airway obstruction. At the end of this chapter, the reader should be able to:

- Describe the characteristic pathology and pathogenesis of the major forms of obstructive lung disease
- Explain the mechanisms for airflow obstruction in asthma, chronic bronchitis, and emphysema
- Compare and contrast the changes in pulmonary mechanics, control of breathing and gas exchange in asthma, chronic bronchitis, and emphysema
- Describe the primary medications used in the management of asthma and COPD and outline the basic treatment approach for each problem
- Identify patients with less common forms of obstructive lung disease including alpha-one antitrypsin deficiency and upper airway obstruction

AIRWAY OBSTRUCTION

Increased resistance to airflow can be caused by conditions (1) inside the airway lumen, (2) in the wall of the airway, and (3) in the peribronchial region (Figure 4.1):

1. The lumen may be partially occluded by excessive secretions, as in chronic bronchitis. Partial obstruction can also occur acutely in pulmonary edema or due to aspirated foreign material or retained secretions. Inhaled foreign bodies may cause localized partial or complete obstruction.

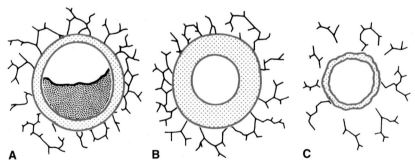

A   **B**   **C**

Figure 4.1. Mechanisms of airway obstruction. A. The lumen is partly blocked, for example, by excessive secretions. **B.** The airway wall is thickened, for example, by edema or hypertrophy of smooth muscle. **C.** The abnormality is outside the airway; in this example, the lung parenchyma is partly destroyed, and the airway has narrowed because of the loss of radial traction.

2. Causes in the wall of the airway include contraction of bronchial smooth muscle, as in asthma; hypertrophy of the mucous glands, as in chronic bronchitis (see Figure 4.6); and inflammation and edema of the wall, as in chronic bronchitis and asthma.
3. Outside the airway, destruction of lung parenchyma may cause loss of radial traction and consequent airway narrowing, as in emphysema. A bronchus may also be compressed an enlarged lymph node or neoplasm external to the airway. Peribronchial edema can also cause narrowing (see Figure 6.5).

CHRONIC OBSTRUCTIVE PULMONARY DISEASE

Chronic obstructive pulmonary disease (COPD) is a syndrome caused by emphysema, chronic bronchitis, or a mixture of the two and is defined by the presence of airflow obstruction, chronic respiratory symptoms, and a risk factor such as smoking or exposure to air pollution. Patients typically have increasing shortness of breath over several years, chronic cough, impaired exercise tolerance, as well as overinflated lungs and impaired gas exchange. Because it can often be difficult to determine to what extent emphysema or chronic bronchitis contributes to the patient's symptoms and pathophysiological derangements, a diagnosis of COPD is more commonly used in clinical practice.

Emphysema

Emphysema is characterized by enlargement of the air spaces distal to the terminal bronchiole, with destruction of their walls. Note that this is an anatomic definition; in other words, the diagnosis is presumptive and based largely on radiologic findings in the living patient.

Pathology
A typical histologic appearance is shown in Figure 4.2. Note that, in contrast to the normal lung section in Figure 4.2A, the emphysematous lung (Figure 4.2B) shows loss of alveolar walls with consequent destruction of parts of the capillary bed. Strands of parenchyma that contain blood vessels can sometimes be seen coursing across large dilated airspaces. The small airways (less than 2 mm wide) are narrowed, tortuous, and reduced in number. In addition, they have thin, atrophied walls. There is also some loss of larger airways. The structural changes are well seen with the naked eye or hand lens in large slices of lung (Figure 4.3).

Types
Various types of emphysema are recognized. The definition given earlier indicates that the disease affects the parenchyma distal to the terminal bronchiole.

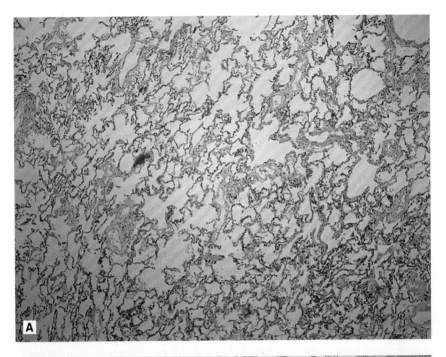

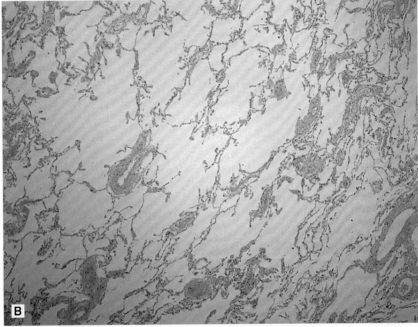

Figure 4.2. Microscopic appearance of emphysematous lung. A. Normal lung.
B. Loss of alveolar walls and consequent enlargement of airspaces (×4). (Image courtesy of Corinne Fligner, MD.)

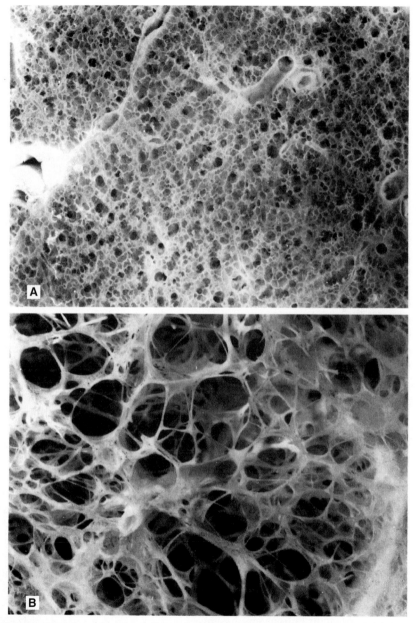

Figure 4.3. Appearance of slices of normal and emphysematous lung. A. Normal.
B. Panacinar emphysema (barium sulfate impregnation, ×14). (Reprinted from Heard BE.
Pathology of Chronic Bronchitis and Emphysema. London, UK: Churchill; 1969. Copyright
© 1969 Elsevier. With permission.)

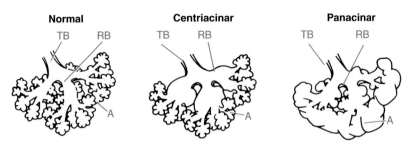

Figure 4.4. Centriacinar and panacinar emphysema. In centriacinar emphysema, the destruction is confined to the terminal and respiratory bronchioles (*TB* and *RB*). In panacinar emphysema, the peripheral alveoli (*A*) are also involved.

This unit is the *acinus*, but it may not be damaged uniformly. In *centriacinar emphysema*, the destruction is limited to the central part of the lobule, and the peripheral alveolar ducts and alveoli may escape unscathed (Figure 4.4). By contrast, *panacinar emphysema* shows distension and destruction of the whole lobule. Occasionally, the disease is most marked in the lung adjacent to interlobular septa (paraseptal emphysema), while in other cases, large cystic areas or bullae develop (bullous emphysema).

Centriacinar and panacinar emphysema tend to have different topographic distributions. The former is typically most marked in the apex of the upper lobe but spreads down the lung as the disease progresses (Figure 4.5A). The predilection for the apex might reflect the higher mechanical stresses (see Figure 3.3), which predispose to structural failure of the alveolar walls. By contrast, panacinar emphysema has no regional preference or, possibly, is more common in the lower lobes. When emphysema is severe, it is difficult to distinguish the two types, and these may coexist in one lung. The centriacinar form is a very common form and is most often due to long-standing exposure to cigarette smoke.

A severe form of panacinar emphysema can be seen in α_1-antitrypsin deficiency (Figure 4.5B). The disease, which usually begins in the lower lobes, may become evident by the age of 40 years in patients who are homozygous for the Z-gene, particularly in those who also smoke. Extrapulmonary manifestations may also be present in the liver, bowel, kidneys, and other organs. Therapy by replacement of α_1-antitrypsin is now available. Heterozygotes do not seem to be at risk, although this is not certain. Other less common variants of emphysema include unilateral emphysema (MacLeod's or Swyer-James syndrome), which causes a unilaterally hyperlucent chest radiograph, and idiopathic giant bullous emphysema.

Pathogenesis
One hypothesis is that excessive amounts of the enzyme lysosomal elastase are released from the neutrophils in the lung. This results in the destruction of elastin, an important structural protein of the lung. Neutrophil

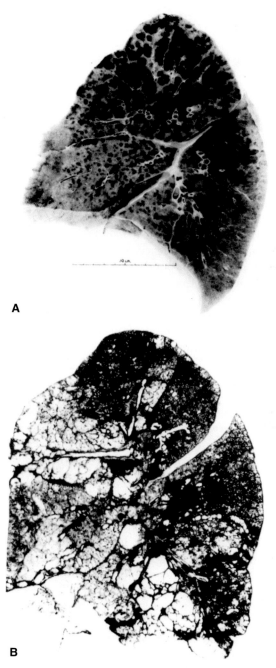

Figure 4.5. **Topographic distribution of emphysema. A.** The typical upper zone preference of centriacinar emphysema. **B.** The typical lower zone preference of emphysema caused by α_1-antitrypsin deficiency. (Reprinted from Heard BE. *Pathology of Chronic Bronchitis and Emphysema*. London, UK: Churchill; 1969. Copyright © 1969 Elsevier. With permission.)

elastase also cleaves type IV collagen, a molecule that contributes to the strength of the thin side of the pulmonary capillary and therefore the integrity of the alveolar wall. Animals that have had neutrophil elastase instilled into their airways develop histologic changes that are similar in many ways to emphysema.

Cigarette smoking is an important pathogenic factor and may work by stimulating macrophages to release neutrophil chemoattractants, such as C5a, or by reducing the activity of elastase inhibitors. In addition, many neutrophils are normally marginated (trapped) in the lung, and this process is exaggerated by cigarette smoking, which also activates trapped leucocytes. This hypothesis puts the etiology on the same footing as that for the emphysema of α_1-antitrypsin deficiency, in which the mechanism is the lack of the antiprotease that normally inhibits elastase. One puzzle is why some heavy smokers do not develop the disease.

Air pollution may play a role, as may hereditary factors, which are clearly important in α_1-antitrypsin deficiency. Smoke pollution from, for example, use of wood-burning stoves in poorly ventilated indoor spaces, is now also recognized as an important cause of COPD worldwide. Whether electronic cigarettes cause emphysema is not clear yet, but evidence from bronchoalveolar lavage studies in users of combustible and electronic cigarettes suggests that electronic cigarette use causes similar disruptions in the protease–antiprotease balance as combustible tobacco.

Chronic Bronchitis

This disease is characterized by excessive mucus production in the bronchial tree, sufficient to cause excessive expectoration of sputum. Unlike the definition of emphysema, this is a clinical definition based on the history obtained from the patient. In practice, criteria for a diagnosis of chronic bronchitis include expectoration of sputum on most days for at least 3 months in the year for at least 2 successive years.

Pathology

The hallmark is hypertrophy of mucous glands in the large bronchi (Figure 4.6) and evidence of chronic inflammatory changes in the small airways. The mucous gland enlargement may be expressed as the gland–wall ratio, referred to as the "Reid index." Normally less than 0.4, this value may exceed 0.7 in severe chronic bronchitis (Figure 4.7). Excessive amounts of mucus are found in the airways, and semisolid plugs of mucus may occlude some small bronchi.

In addition, the small airways are narrowed and show inflammatory changes, including cellular infiltration and edema of the walls. Granulation tissue is present, bronchial smooth muscle increases, and peribronchial fibrosis may develop. There is evidence that the initial pathologic changes are in the small airways and that these progress to the larger bronchi.

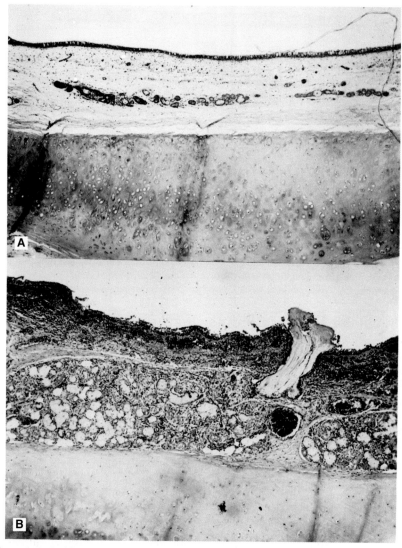

Figure 4.6. Histologic changes in chronic bronchitis. A. A normal bronchial wall. **B.** Bronchial wall of a patient with chronic bronchitis. Note the great hypertrophy of the mucous glands, the thickened submucosa, and the cellular infiltration (3 × 60). Compare with the diagram of the bronchial wall in Figure 4.7. (Reprinted from Thurlbeck WM. *Chronic Airflow Obstruction in Lung Disease.* Philadelphia, PA: WB Saunders; 1976. Copyright © 1976 Elsevier. With permission.)

Pathogenesis

As with emphysema, cigarette smoking is the primary cause, as repeated exposure to this inhaled irritant results in chronic inflammation. Air pollution caused by smog or industrial or household smoke is another definite factor.

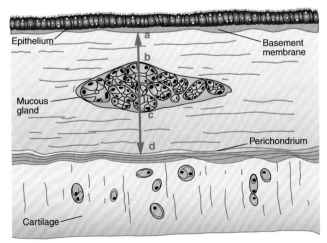

Figure 4.7. **Structure of a normal bronchial wall**. In chronic bronchitis, the thickness of the mucous glands increases and can be expressed as the Reid index given by (b–c)/(a–d). (Reprinted from Thurlbeck WM. *Chronic Airflow Obstruction in Lung Disease*. Philadelphia, PA: WB Saunders; 1976. Copyright © 1976 Elsevier. With permission.)

Clinical Features of Chronic Obstructive Pulmonary Disease

Because chronic bronchitis is defined clinically, the diagnosis can be made confidently in the living patient. The extent of emphysema in a given patient is uncertain; however. Definitive diagnosis requires histologic confirmation that is usually not available during life, although a combination of findings on physical examination and chest imaging can indicate a high probability of the diagnosis. This is why COPD is the more commonly used term in clinical practice.

Within the spectrum of COPD, two extremes of clinical presentation have been recognized: type A and type B. At one time, it was thought that these types correlated to some extent with the relative amounts of emphysema and chronic bronchitis, respectively, but this view has been challenged and, in practice, most patients have features of both. Nevertheless, it is still useful to describe two patterns of clinical presentation because they represent different pathophysiologies.

Type A

A typical presentation would be a patient in their middle 50s who has had increasing shortness of breath for the last 3 or 4 years. Cough may be absent or may produce little white sputum. Physical examination reveals an asthenic build with evidence of recent weight loss. There is no cyanosis. The chest is overexpanded with quiet breath sounds and no adventitious sounds. The radiograph (Figure 4.8B) confirms the overinflation with low and flattened diaphragms, narrow mediastinum, and increased retrosternal translucency (between the sternum and the heart on the lateral view). In addition, the radiograph shows increased lucency, particularly in the apical lung zones, due to attenuation and narrowing of the peripheral pulmonary vessels. Additional information is available from computer tomography (CT). Figure 4.9A shows a normal lung, while Figure 4.9B shows an example of emphysema, denoted by the large holes scattered throughout the lung. These patients have been referred to in the past as "pink puffers," although this term has fallen out of clinical practice.

Type B

A typical presentation would be a patient in their 50s with a history of chronic productive cough over several years. The expectoration gradually increases in

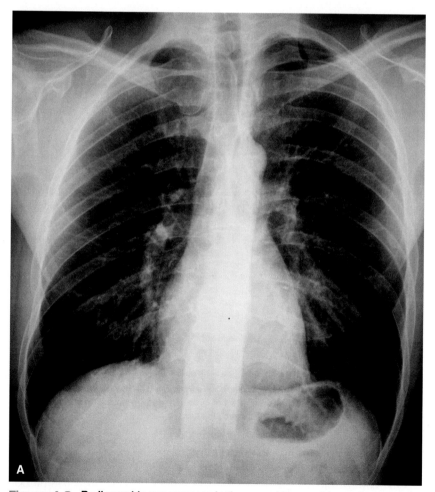

Figure 4.8. **Radiographic appearances in the normal lung and in emphysema.**
A. Normal lung.

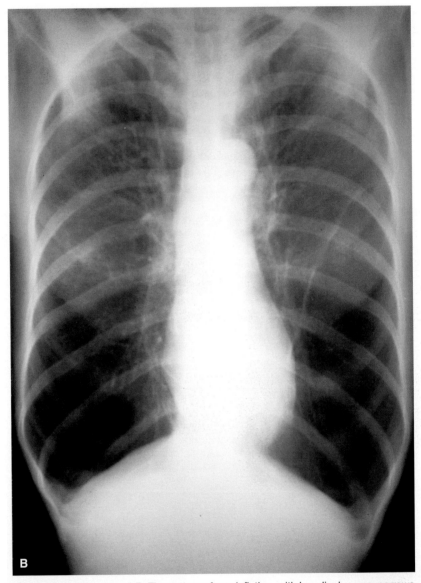

B

Figure 4.8. *(Continued)* **B.** The pattern of overinflation, with low diaphragms, narrows mediastinum, and increased translucency that is seen in emphysema. The emphysema is particularly prominent in the lower regions of the lung.

severity, being present only in the winter months initially but, as the disease progresses, lasting most of the year.

On examination, the patient has a stocky build with a plethoric complexion and some cyanosis. Auscultation reveals scattered rales (crackles) and rhonchi (whistles). There may be signs of fluid retention with a raised jugular venous

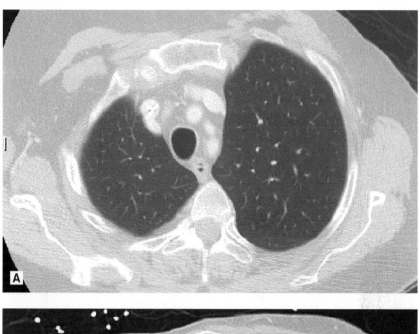

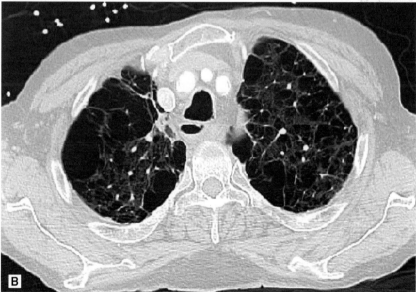

Figure 4.9. **A.** Appearance of normal lung on CT scan of the chest. **B.** CT scan of the lungs of a patient with emphysema. Holes can be seen scattered throughout the lung.

pressure and ankle edema. The chest radiograph shows some cardiac enlargement, congested lung fields, and increased markings attributable to old infection. Parallel lines (tram lines) may be seen, probably caused by the thickened walls of inflamed bronchi. At autopsy, chronic inflammatory changes in the bronchi are the rule if the patient had severe bronchitis, but there may be severe emphysema as well. These patients have been referred to in the past as "blue bloaters." This term has also fallen out of clinical practice.

Both the Type A and Type B patients have shortness of breath on exertion that worsens over time and progressively limits exercise tolerance. These patients are almost invariably cigarette smokers of many years' duration, which can be quantified as the number of cigarette packs a day multiplied by the number of years of smoking to give the "pack-years." Both groups of patients are at risk for exacerbations in which they experience significant worsening of their chronic, daily symptoms, which prompt more urgent evaluation in the clinic or hospital.

Some physicians believe that the essential difference between the two types is in the control of breathing. They suggest that the more severe hypoxemia and consequent higher incidence of cor pulmonale in the type B patients can be attributed to a reduced ventilatory drive, especially during sleep.

Features of Type A and Type B Presentations in COPD

Type A	Type B
Increasing dyspnea over years	Increasing dyspnea over years
Little or no cough	Frequent cough with sputum
Marked chest overexpansion	Moderate or no increase in chest volume
No cyanosis	Often cyanosis
Quiet breath sounds	Rales and rhonchi
Normal jugular venous pressure	Raised jugular venous pressure
No peripheral edema	Peripheral edema
Arterial P_{O_2} only moderately depressed	P_{O_2} often very low
Arterial P_{CO_2} normal	P_{CO_2} often increased

Pulmonary Function

Most of the features of disordered function in COPD follow from the pathologic features discussed earlier and illustrated in Figures 4.2 to 4.7.

Ventilatory Capacity and Mechanics

The forced expiratory volume in 1 second (FEV_1), forced vital capacity (FVC), forced expiratory volume as a percentage of vital capacity (FEV_1/FVC), forced expiratory flow ($FEF_{25\%-75\%}$), and maximum expiratory flow at 50% and 75% of exhaled vital capacity ($\dot{V}max_{50\%}$ and $\dot{V}max_{75\%}$) are all reduced. All of these measurements reflect the airway obstruction, whether caused by excessive mucus in the lumen, thickening of the wall by inflammatory changes (see Figure 4.1A and B), or by the loss of radial traction (see Figure 4.1C). The FVC is reduced because the airways close prematurely during expiration at an abnormally high lung volume, giving an increased residual volume (RV).

Examination of the spirogram shows that the flow rate over most of the forced expiration is greatly reduced, and the *expiratory time* is increased. Indeed, some physicians regard this prolonged time as a useful simple bedside index of obstruction. Often, the maneuver is terminated by breathlessness when the patient is still exhaling. The low flow rate over most of the forced expiration partly reflects the reduced elastic recoil of the emphysematous lung, which generates the pressure responsible for flow under these conditions of dynamic compression (see Figure 1.6). In severe disease, the FEV_1 may be reduced to less than 1.0 liter whereas healthy young individuals may have values at or above 4 liters depending on their age, height, and sex (see Appendix A).

In some patients, the FEV_1, FVC, and FEV_1/FVC may increase significantly after the administration of a short-acting bronchodilator, such as albuterol, although the airflow obstruction is incompletely reversible. Significant response to bronchodilators suggests asthma, which can overlap with COPD.

The expiratory flow–volume curve is also grossly abnormal in severe disease. Figure 1.8 shows that, after a brief interval of moderately high flow, flow is strikingly reduced as the airways collapse, and flow limitation by dynamic compression occurs. The graphed curve often has a scooped-out appearance. Flow is greatly reduced in relation to lung volume and ceases at a high lung volume because of premature airway closure (see Figure 1.5B). However, the inspiratory flow–volume curve may be normal or nearly so (see Figure 1.9) as the airways are tethered open by radial traction exerted by the surrounding alveolar walls during inhalation.

The total lung capacity (TLC), functional residual capacity (FRC), and RV are all typically increased in emphysema. Often, the RV/TLC ratio may exceed 0.4 (less than 0.3 in young healthy individuals). There is often a striking discrepancy between the FRC determined by the body plethysmograph and by the gas dilution techniques (helium equilibration), the former being higher by 1 liter or more. This may be caused by regions of uncommunicating lung behind grossly distorted airways. However, the disparity more often reflects the slow equilibration process in poorly ventilated areas. These static lung volumes are also often abnormal in patients with chronic bronchitis, although the increases in volume are generally less marked.

Elastic recoil of the lung is reduced in emphysema (see Figure 3.1), the pressure–volume curve being displaced up and to the left. This change reflects the disorganization and loss of elastic tissue as a result of the destruction of alveolar walls. The transpulmonary pressure at TLC is low. In uncomplicated chronic bronchitis in the absence of emphysema, the pressure–volume curve may be nearly normal because the parenchyma is little affected.

Airway resistance related to lung volume is increased in COPD due to all of the factors shown in Figure 4.1. However, it is possible to distinguish between an increased resistance caused by intrinsic narrowing of the airway walls or debris in the lumen (Figure 4.1A and B) and the loss of elastic recoil and radial traction (Figure 4.1C). This can be done by relating resistance

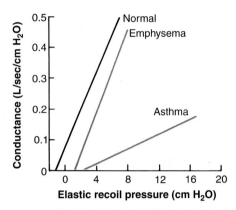

Figure 4.10. **Relationships between airway conductance and elastic recoil pressure in obstructive pulmonary disease.** Note that the line for emphysema lies close to the normal line. It is evident that any increase in airway resistance is chiefly caused by the smaller elastic recoil of the lung. By contrast, in asthma, the line is markedly abnormal due to the intrinsic narrowing of the airways. (Reprinted from Colebatch HJH, Finucane KE, Smith MM. Pulmonary conductance and elastic recoil relationships in asthma and emphysema. *J Appl Physiol.* 1973;34(2):143–153. Copyright © 1973 by American Physiological Society (APS). All rights reserved.)

to the static elastic recoil. Figure 4.10 shows airway conductance (reciprocal of resistance) plotted against static transpulmonary pressure in a series of 10 healthy patients, 10 patients with emphysema (without bronchitis), and 10 patients with asthma. The measurements were made during a quiet, unforced expiration. Note that the relationship between conductance and transpulmonary pressure for the patients with emphysema was almost normal. In other words, we can ascribe their reduced ventilatory capacity almost entirely to the effects of the smaller elastic recoil pressure of the lung. This not only reduces the effective driving pressure during a forced expiration but also allows the airways to collapse more easily because of the loss of radial traction. The small displacement of the emphysematous line to the right probably reflects the distortion and loss of airways in this disease.

By contrast, the line for the patients with asthma shows that the airway conductance was greatly reduced at a given recoil pressure. Thus, the higher resistance in these patients can be ascribed to intrinsic narrowing of the airways caused by contraction of smooth muscle and inflammatory changes in the airways. Although not shown in Figure 4.10, administration of a bronchodilating medication would move the line toward the normal position. Comparable data are not available for a group of patients with chronic bronchitis without emphysema because it is virtually impossible to select such a group during life. However, Figure 4.10 clarifies the behavior of different types of airway obstruction.

Gas Exchange

Ventilation–perfusion inequality is inevitable in COPD and leads to hypoxemia with or without CO_2 retention. Typically, the type A patient has only moderate hypoxemia (P_{O_2} often in the high 60s or 70s), with a normal arterial P_{CO_2}. By contrast, the type B patient often has severe hypoxemia (P_{O_2} often in the 50s or 40s) with an increased P_{CO_2}, especially in advanced disease.

The alveolar–arterial P_{O_2} difference is always increased, especially in patients with severe chronic bronchitis. An analysis based on the concept of the ideal point (see Figure 2.7) reveals increases in both physiologic dead space and physiologic shunt. The dead space is particularly increased in emphysema, whereas high values for physiologic shunt are especially common in chronic bronchitis.

The reasons for these differences are clarified by the results obtained with the inert gas elimination technique. First, review Figure 2.8, which shows a typical pattern in a normal subject. By contrast, Figure 4.11 shows a typical distribution in a patient with advanced type A disease. This 76-year-old man had a history of increasing dyspnea over several years. The chest radiograph showed hyperinflation with attenuated small pulmonary vessels. The arterial P_{O_2} and P_{CO_2} were 68 and 39 mm Hg, respectively.

The distribution shows that a large amount of ventilation went to lung units with high ventilation–perfusion ratios ($\dot{V}_A/\dot{Q}$) (compare Figure 2.8). This would be shown as physiologic dead space in the ideal point analysis, and the excessive ventilation is largely wasted from the point of view of gas exchange. By contrast, there is little blood flow to units with an abnormally low $\dot{V}_A/\dot{Q}$. This explains the relatively mild degree of hypoxemia in the patient and the fact that the calculated physiologic shunt was only slightly increased.

These findings can be contrasted with those shown in Figure 4.12, which shows the distribution in a 47-year-old man with advanced chronic bronchitis and type B disease. The arterial P_{O_2} and P_{CO_2} were 47 and 50 mm Hg, respectively. Note that there was some increase in ventilation to high $\dot{V}_A/\dot{Q}$ units (physiologic dead space). However, the distribution chiefly shows large

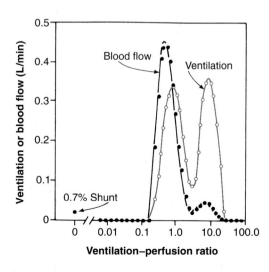

Figure 4.11. Distribution of ventilation–perfusion ratios in a patient with type A COPD. Note the large amount of ventilation to units with high ventilation–perfusion ratios (physiologic dead space). (Republished with permission of the American Society for Clinical Investigation, from Wagner PD, Dantzker DR, Dueck R, et al. Ventilation–perfusion inequality in chronic pulmonary disease. *J Clin Invest.* 1977;59(2):203–216; permission conveyed through Copyright Clearance Center, Inc.)

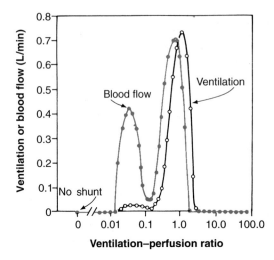

Figure 4.12. Distribution of ventilation–perfusion ratios in a patient with type B COPD. There is a large amount of blood flow to units with low ventilation–perfusion ratios (physiologic shunt). (Republished with permission of the American Society for Clinical Investigation, from Wagner PD, Dantzker DR, Dueck R, et al. Ventilation–perfusion inequality in chronic pulmonary disease. *J Clin Invest.* 1977;59(2):203–216; permission conveyed through Copyright Clearance Center, Inc.)

amounts of blood flow to low $\dot{V}_A/\dot{Q}$ units (physiologic shunt), accounting for his severe hypoxemia. It is remarkable that there was no blood flow to unventilated alveoli (true shunt). Indeed, true shunts of more than a few percent are uncommon in COPD. Note that although the patterns shown in Figures 4.11 and 4.12 are typical, considerable variation is seen in patients with COPD.

On exercise, the arterial P_{O_2} may fall or rise depending on the response of the ventilation and the cardiac output and the changes in the distribution of ventilation and blood flow. In some patients at least, the main factor in the fall of P_{O_2} is the limited cardiac output, which exaggerates hypoxemia in the presence of ventilation–perfusion inequality. Patients with CO_2 retention often show higher P_{CO_2} values on exercise because of their limited ventilatory capacity and inability to eliminate CO_2 produced in the exercising muscles.

The reasons for the ventilation–perfusion inequality are clear when we consider the disorganization of the lung architecture in emphysema (Figures 4.2 and 4.3) and the abnormalities in airways in chronic bronchitis (Figure 4.6). There is ample evidence of uneven ventilation as determined by the single-breath nitrogen washout (see Figure 1.10). In addition, topographic measurements with radioactive materials show regional inequality of both ventilation and blood flow. The blood flow inequality is largely caused by the destruction of portions of the capillary bed.

The deleterious effects of airway obstruction on gas exchange are reduced by collateral ventilation that occurs in these patients. Communicating channels normally exist between adjacent alveoli and between neighboring small airways, and there have been many experimental demonstrations of these. The fact that there is so little blood flow to unventilated units in these patients (Figures 4.11 and 4.12) emphasizes the effectiveness of collateral ventilation because some airways must presumably be completely obstructed, especially in severe bronchitis.

Another factor that reduces the amount of ventilation–perfusion inequality is hypoxic pulmonary vasoconstriction. (See *West's Respiratory Physiology: The Essentials*, 11th ed., p. 56-57.) This local response to a low alveolar P_{O_2} reduces the blood flow to poorly ventilated and unventilated regions, minimizing the arterial hypoxemia. When patients with COPD are given bronchodilators, such as albuterol, they sometimes develop a slight fall in arterial P_{O_2}. This is probably caused by the vasodilator action of these β-adrenergic drugs, increasing the blood flow to poorly ventilated areas. This finding is more marked in asthma (see Figures 4.17 and 4.18).

The arterial P_{CO_2} is often normal in patients with mild to moderate COPD despite their ventilation–perfusion inequality. Any tendency for the arterial P_{CO_2} to rise stimulates the chemoreceptors, thus increasing ventilation to the alveoli (see Figure 2.9). As the disease becomes more severe, the arterial P_{CO_2} may rise. This is particularly likely to occur in type B patients. The increased work of breathing is an important factor, but there is also evidence that the sensitivity of the respiratory center to CO_2 is reduced in some of these patients.

If the arterial P_{CO_2} rises, the pH tends to fall, resulting in respiratory acidosis. Because the P_{CO_2} rises slowly over time, the kidney can compensate adequately by retaining bicarbonate, and the pH remains almost normal (compensated respiratory acidosis). The P_{CO_2} may rise more suddenly during COPD exacerbations or acute chest infections, leading to acute respiratory acidosis (see Chapter 8, Respiratory Failure).

Additional information about gas exchange in these patients can be obtained by measuring the diffusing capacity (transfer factor) for carbon monoxide (see Figure 2.12). The diffusing capacity as measured by the single-breath method is particularly likely to be reduced in patients with severe emphysema due to the loss of surface area that occurs with enlargement of the airspaces. By contrast, patients with chronic bronchitis but little parenchymal destruction may have normal values.

Pulmonary Circulation

The pulmonary artery pressure frequently rises in patients with COPD as their disease progresses. Several factors are responsible. In emphysema, large portions of the capillary bed are destroyed, thus increasing vascular resistance. Hypoxic pulmonary vasoconstriction also raises the pulmonary arterial pressure. Additional increases can be seen during exacerbations due to worsening alveolar hypoxia and/or respiratory acidosis. In advanced disease, histologic changes in the walls of the small arteries occur. Finally, these patients often develop polycythemia as a response to the hypoxemia, thus increasing blood viscosity. This occurs most commonly in patients with severe bronchitis, who tend to have the lowest arterial P_{O_2}.

Fluid retention with dependent edema and engorged neck veins may occur, especially in type B patients. The right heart often enlarges with characteristic radiologic and electrocardiographic appearances. Changes in the structure and/or function of the right ventricle as a result of chronic lung disease are termed "cor pulmonale." The output of the heart may actually be increased because it is operating high on the Starling curve, and the output can rise further on exercise.

Control of Ventilation

As indicated previously, some patients with COPD develop CO_2 retention because they do not sufficiently maintain ventilation to their alveoli. The reasons why some patients behave in this way and some do not are not completely understood. One factor is the increased work of breathing due to the high airway resistance, which markedly increases the O_2 cost of breathing (Figure 4.13). Normal subjects have an abnormally small ventilatory response to inhaled CO_2 if they are asked to breathe through a high resistance. Thus, a patient with a severely limited O_2 consumption may be willing to forgo a normal arterial P_{CO_2} to obtain the advantage of a reduced work of breathing and a correspondingly reduced O_2 cost. However, the correlation between airway resistance and arterial P_{CO_2} is sufficiently poor that some other factor must be involved.

Measurements of the ventilatory response to inhaled CO_2 show that there are significant differences among normal subjects. These differences are partly caused by genetic factors. Some patients have a reduced respiratory center output in response to inhaled CO_2, many have a mechanical obstruction to ventilation, and some patients have both. Thus, it is possible that the ventilatory response of a patient in the face of severe ventilation–perfusion inequality and increased work of breathing is predetermined to some extent by these factors.

Changes in Early Disease

So far, we have been concerned mainly with pulmonary function in patients with well-established disease. However, relatively little can be done to reverse

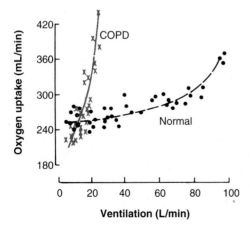

Figure 4.13. Oxygen uptake during voluntary hyperventilation in patients with COPD. Note the high values compared with those of the normal subjects. (Reprinted from Cherniack RM, Cherniack L, Naimark A. *Respiration in Health and Disease.* 2nd ed. Philadelphia, PA: WB Saunders, 1972. Copyright © 1972 Elsevier. With permission.)

the disease process in this group, and the treatment is limited chiefly to symptom relief with bronchodilators, prevention and control of infection, and pulmonary rehabilitation programs. There has long been interest in identifying patients with early disease in the hope that the changes can be arrested or reversed by elimination of smoking or other risk factors such as exposure to pollution.

It was emphasized in Chapter 1 that because relatively little of the airway resistance resides in small airways (less than 2 mm wide), pathophysiologic changes there may go unnoticed by the usual pulmonary function tests. Given evidence that the earliest changes in COPD occur in these small airways, interest has focused on whether changes in parameters that reflect small airways function including the $FEF_{25\%-75\%}$, $\dot{V}max_{50\%}$, $\dot{V}max_{75\%}$ and closing volume can be used to identify such early disease. Unfortunately, studies have not supported a role in this regard, and we still lack effective ways to identify people at risk for progressing COPD at an early, asymptomatic stage.

Treatment of Patients with COPD

Smoking cessation is the most critical step for most patients, as this is the one intervention that can slow the rate of decline in lung function over time. Exposure to occupational, atmospheric, and household pollution should also be reduced as far as possible. Bronchodilator therapy, including beta-agonists and antimuscarinics, are the mainstay of therapy for all patients with chronic, stable COPD, with the intensity of use varying depending on the severity of the patient's airflow obstruction, functional limitation, and frequency of exacerbations. Inhaled corticosteroids are also used in many patients but are generally reserved for those with more severe disease and/or frequent exacerbations, while the macrolide antibiotic, azithromycin, and phosphodiesterase-4 inhibitor, roflumilast, are sometimes used on a chronic basis in patients who suffer from frequent exacerbations. Pulmonary rehabilitation can be prescribed to patients with stable disease of any severity and has been shown to quality of life and exercise capacity. Administration of continuous supplemental oxygen to patients with sufficient degrees of chronic hypoxemia is associated with improved survival in such patients. One benefit of this intervention is an increase in the average alveolar P_{O_2}, which lessens hypoxic pulmonary vasoconstriction and partially alleviates the pulmonary hypertension. Exacerbations of COPD are managed with systemically delivered corticosteroids, aggressive use of short-acting bronchodilators and, when indicated, mechanical ventilatory support.

Lung Volume Reduction Surgery

Surgery to reduce the volume of the overexpanded lung can be valuable in selected cases. The aim is to remove emphysematous and avascular areas and to preserve the nearly normal regions. The physiologic basis is that reducing the volume increases the radial traction on the airways and therefore helps to limit dynamic airway compression. In addition, the inspiratory muscles, particularly the diaphragm, are shortened with consequent improvement in their mechanical efficiency. Criteria for surgery usually include an FEV_1 of less than 45% predicted, lung volume measurements consistent with air trapping and hyperinflation, upper lobe–predominant emphysema demonstrated by CT scan and low exercise capacity following a pulmonary rehabilitation program. In properly selected patients, lung volume reduction surgery (LVRS) is associated with improvements in spirometry, lung volumes, quality of life, and dyspnea and, in a small set of patients, improved survival.

ASTHMA

This disease is characterized by inflammation and increased responsiveness of the airways to various stimuli and is manifested as widespread narrowing of the airways that change in severity, either spontaneously or as a result of treatment.

Pathology

The airways have hypertrophied smooth muscle that contracts during an attack, causing bronchoconstriction (Figure 4.1B). In addition, there is hypertrophy of mucous glands, edema of the bronchial wall, and extensive infiltration by eosinophils and lymphocytes (Figure 4.14). The mucus is increased in volume, as well as thick, tenacious, and slow moving. In severe cases, many airways are occluded by mucous plugs, some of which may be coughed up in the sputum. Subepithelial fibrosis is common in patients with chronic asthma and is part of the process called remodeling. In uncomplicated asthma, there is no destruction of alveolar walls, and there are no copious purulent bronchial secretions. Occasionally, the abundance of eosinophils in the sputum gives a purulent appearance, which may be wrongly ascribed to infection.

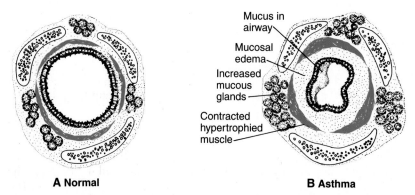

Mucus in airway
Mucosal edema
Increased mucous glands
Contracted hypertrophied muscle

A Normal   **B Asthma**

Figure 4.14. Diagram of the normal bronchial wall (A) and the bronchial wall in asthma (B). Note the hypertrophied, contracted smooth muscle, edema, mucous gland hypertrophy, and secretion in the lumen.

Pathogenesis

Two features that are common to all patients with asthma are airway hyperresponsiveness and airway inflammation. Research suggests that airway inflammation is responsible for all the associated features of asthma, including the increased airway hyperresponsiveness, airway edema, hypersecretion of mucus, and inflammatory cell infiltration. However, a fundamental abnormality of airway smooth muscle or regulation of airway tone is possible in some patients.

Epidemiologic studies indicate that asthma begins in childhood in the majority of cases and that an allergic diathesis often plays an important role. Frequent exposure to typical childhood infections and environments favoring fecal contamination are associated with a lower incidence of asthma. These observations and others have led to the "hygiene hypothesis," which suggests that children in a critical stage of development of the immune response who are not frequently exposed to typical childhood infectious agents may more frequently develop an allergic diathesis and asthma.

It is also clear that environmental factors and atmospheric pollutants play an important role and may be responsible for the increase in the prevalence and severity of asthma over the last 40 years in modernized, affluent western countries. Such factors likely also account for the increased prevalence and worse disease outcomes among underrepresented minority populations in many large cities, who are often disproportionately affected by these environmental factors. There is also a complex interaction between these environmental factors and genetic factors, as linkage analysis has identified a variety of chromosomal loci associated with asthma.

The trigger for the development of airway inflammation cannot always be identified. It is well recognized in some instances, as in the case for some antigens in persons with allergic asthma (Figure 4.15). However, in other types of asthma, such as exercise-induced asthma or asthma following a viral respiratory tract infection, the trigger is not recognized.

A single inflammatory cell type or inflammatory mediator does not appear to be responsible for all manifestations of asthma. Eosinophils, mast cells, neutrophils, lymphocytes, macrophages, and basophils have all been implicated. There is also evidence that noninflammatory cells, including airway epithelial cells and neural cells, especially those of peptidergic nerves, contribute to the inflammation. Some investigators believe that eosinophils play a central effector role in most cases of asthma. There is also evidence that lymphocytes, especially T-cells have an important role, both because they respond to specific antigens and because they modulate inflammatory cell function.

Many inflammatory mediators have been identified in asthma. Cytokines are probably important, particularly those associated with Th-2, helper T-cell activation. These cytokines include interleukin-3 (IL-3), IL-4, IL-5, and IL-13. It is believed that these cytokines are at least partly responsible for modulating inflammatory and immune cell function and for supporting

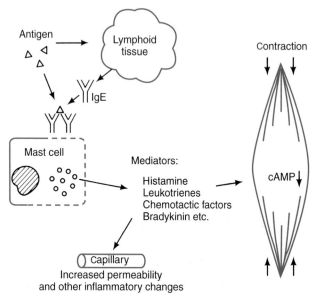

Figure 4.15. Some pathogenic changes in allergic asthma. (See text for details.)

the inflammatory response in the airway. Other inflammatory mediators that probably play a role, particularly in acute bronchoconstriction, include arachidonic acid metabolites, such as leukotrienes and prostaglandins, platelet-activating factor (PAF), neuropeptides, reactive oxygen species, kinins, histamine, and adenosine.

Clinical Features

Asthma commonly begins in children but may occur at any age. In all individuals with asthma, there is general hyperreactivity of the airways, with the result that allergens or nonspecific irritants, such as smoke, cold air, and exercise cause symptoms. Some patients have a previous history to suggest atopy, including allergic rhinitis, eczema, or urticaria, and may relate increases in symptoms to a specific allergen, for example, ragweed or cats. Such a patient is said to have allergic asthma. Many such patients have an increased total serum IgE, increased specific IgE, and peripheral blood eosinophils. Aspirin ingestion is a cause in some individuals because of inhibition of the cyclooxygenase pathway. If there is no general history of allergy and no external allergen can be identified, the term "nonallergic asthma" is used.

For many patients, asthma is an episodic disease with periods of no or well-controlled symptoms, punctuated by periods of worsening disease control. Other patients, however, have more persistent symptoms and require daily medications. When symptomatic, patients may have one, some or all of the cardinal symptoms of asthma, including dyspnea, chest tightness, wheezing, and cough. All patients with asthma are at risk for exacerbations, periods of markedly worsening symptoms that can, in some cases, be life-threatening. Often referred to as "asthma attacks," exacerbations may follow changes in air quality or viral infections, but can also occur without obvious triggers. During an attack, the patient may be extremely dyspneic, orthopneic, and anxious and complain of chest tightness. The accessory muscles of respiration are active and wheezes can be heard in all lung fields. The pulse is rapid, and pulsus paradoxus, a marked fall in systolic and pulse pressure during inspiration, may be present. The sputum is scant and viscid. The chest radiograph reveals hyperinflation but is otherwise without opacities. *Status asthmaticus* refers to an attack that continues for hours or even days without remission despite bronchodilator and corticosteroid therapy. There are often signs of exhaustion, dehydration, and marked tachycardia. The chest may become ominously silent, and vigorous treatment is urgently required. Death can occur in severe exacerbations, often as a result of respiratory failure or cardiovascular collapse due to severe air trapping and its subsequent adverse effects on venous return and cardiac preload.

Diagnosis

The diagnosis of asthma is confirmed by demonstrating reversible airflow obstruction. This is commonly done by documenting a bronchodilator response on spirometry. Because spirometry can be normal during periods of absent symptoms, other strategies include demonstrating temporal changes in spirometry relative to changes in symptoms or demonstrating sufficient variability in peak expiratory flow over time. When the diagnosis is uncertain, the hyperreactivity (or hyperresponsiveness) of the airways can be tested by exposing the patient to increasing inhaled doses of methacholine and measuring the FEV_1. The dose that results in a 20% fall in FEV_1 is known as the PD_{20} (provocative dose 20). Airway hyperresponsiveness can also be tested by measuring spirometry before and after specially designed exercise protocols and demonstrating a decrease in FEV_1 in the postexercise period.

Pulmonary Function

As was the case with chronic bronchitis and emphysema, the changes in lung function generally follow clearly from the pathology of asthma. These changes may be absent or small in magnitude when symptoms are absent but quite marked during exacerbations.

Ventilatory Capacity and Mechanics

During periods of worsening disease control, all indices of expiratory flow rate are reduced significantly, including the FEV_1, FEV_1/FVC, $FEF_{25\%-75\%}$, $\dot{V}max_{50\%}$, and $\dot{V}max_{75\%}$. The FVC is also usually reduced because airways close prematurely toward the end of a full expiration. Between attacks, some

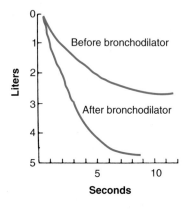

Figure 4.16. Examples of forced expirations before and after bronchodilator therapy in a patient with bronchial asthma. Note the striking increase in flow rate and vital capacity. (Reprinted from Bates DV, Macklem PT, Christie RV. *Respiratory Function in Disease.* 2nd ed. Philadelphia, PA: WB Saunders, 1971. Copyright © 1971 Elsevier. With permission.)

impairment of ventilatory capacity can usually be demonstrated, although the patient may report no symptoms and have a normal physical exam. Typically, all indices increase substantially when a short-acting bronchodilator, such as albuterol, is administered to a patient during an attack, and the change is a valuable measure of the responsiveness of the airways (Figure 4.16). The extent of the increase varies according to the severity of the disease. In status asthmaticus, little change may be seen because the bronchi have become unresponsive (although pulmonary function tests are rarely measured during such acute presentations). Patients in remission may show only minor improvement following bronchodilator administration, although generally there is some.

There is some evidence that the relative change in FEV_1 and FVC after bronchodilator therapy indicates whether the bronchospasm has been completely relieved. During an asthma attack, both the FEV_1 and FVC tend to increase by the same fraction, with the result that the FEV_1/FVC remains low and almost constant. However, when the tone of the airway muscle is nearly normal, the FEV_1 responds more than the FVC, and the FEV_1/FVC approaches the normal value of approximately 0.8.

The flow–volume curve in asthma has the typical obstructive pattern, although it may not exhibit the scooped-out appearance seen in emphysema (see Figure 1.8). After a bronchodilator, flows are higher at all lung volumes, and the whole curve may shift as the TLC and RV are reduced.

Static lung volumes are increased, and remarkably high values for FRC and TLC during asthma attacks have been reported. The increased RV is caused by premature airway closure during a full expiration as a result of the increased smooth muscle tone, edema and inflammation of the airway walls, and abnormal secretions. The cause of the increased FRC and TLC is not fully understood. However, there is some loss of elastic recoil, and the pressure–volume curve is shifted upward and to the left (see Figure 3.1). This tends to return toward normal after a bronchodilator has been given. There is some evidence that changes in the surface tension of the alveolar lining layer may be responsible for the altered elastic properties. The rise in lung volume tends to decrease resistance of the airways by increasing their radial traction. The FRC measured by helium dilution is usually considerably below that found with the body plethysmograph, reflecting the presence of occluded airways or the delayed equilibration of poorly ventilated areas.

Airway resistance as measured in the body plethysmograph is raised, and it falls after a bronchodilator. It is likely that the bronchospasm affects airways of all sizes, and the relationship between airway conductance and elastic recoil pressure is significantly abnormal (Figure 4.10). Narrowing of the large- and medium-sized bronchi can be seen directly at bronchoscopy.

Gas Exchange

Hypoxemia is typically not present during periods of good symptom control but can develop during exacerbations as a result of ventilation–perfusion ($\dot{V}_A/\dot{Q}$) inequality. There is ample evidence of uneven ventilation, and measurements with radioactive gases show regions of reduced ventilation. Marked topographical inequality of blood flow is also seen, and, typically, different areas show transient reductions at different times. Both physiologic dead space and physiologic shunt are generally abnormally high.

An example of a distribution of ventilation–perfusion ratios in a 47-year-old individual with asthma is shown in Figure 4.17. This patient had only mild symptoms at the time of the measurement. The distribution is strikingly different from the normal distribution shown in Figure 2.8. Note especially the bimodal distribution with a considerable amount of the total blood flow (approximately 25%) to units with a low $\dot{V}_A/\dot{Q}$ (approximately 0.1).

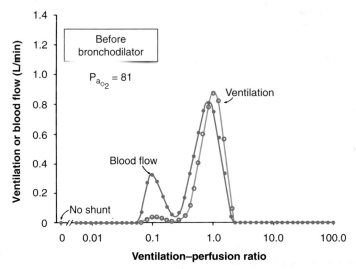

Figure 4.17. Distribution of ventilation–perfusion ratios in a patient with asthma. Note the bimodal appearance, with approximately 25% of the blood flowing to units with ventilation–perfusion ratios in the region of 0.1.

This accounts for the patient's mild hypoxemia, the arterial P_{O_2} being 81 mm Hg. There is no pure shunt (blood flow to unventilated alveoli), a surprising finding in view of the mucous plugging of airways, which is a feature of the disease.

When this patient was given the bronchodilator isoproterenol by aerosol, there was an increase in $FEF_{25\%-75\%}$ from 3.4 to 4.2 L/sec. Thus, there was some relief of his bronchospasm. The changes in the distribution of ventilation–perfusion ratios are shown in Figure 4.18. Note that the blood flow to the low $\dot{V}_A/\dot{Q}$ alveoli increased from approximately 25% to 50% of the flow, resulting in a fall in arterial P_{O_2} from 81 to 70 mm Hg. The mean $\dot{V}_A/\dot{Q}$ of the low mode increased slightly from 0.10 to 0.14, indicating that the ventilation to these units increased slightly more than their blood flow. Again, no shunt was seen. The absence of shunt—that is, blood flow to unventilated lung units—in Figures 4.17 and 4.18 is striking, especially because asthmatics who come to autopsy have mucous plugs in many of their airways. Presumably, the explanation is collateral ventilation that reaches lung situated behind completely closed bronchioles. This is shown diagrammatically in Figure 1.11. The same mechanism probably exists in the lungs of patients with chronic bronchitis (see for example, Figure 4.12).

Bronchodilators can decrease the arterial P_{O_2} in patients with asthma. The mechanism of the increased hypoxemia is apparently relief of vasoconstriction in poorly ventilated areas. This vasoconstriction probably results from the release of mediators, as happens with bronchoconstriction. The fall in P_{O_2} is accompanied by increases in physiologic shunt and dead space. The favorable effects of bronchodilators, such as albuterol, on airway resistance far exceed the disadvantages of the mild additional hypoxemia.

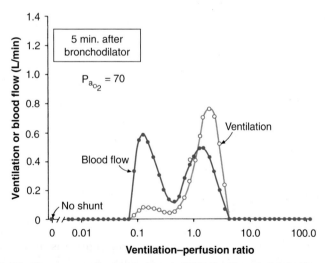

Figure 4.18. The same patient as in Figure 4.17 after the administration of the bronchodilator isoproterenol by aerosol. Note the increase in blood flow to the units with low ventilation–perfusion ratios and the corresponding fall in arterial P_{O_2}.

During periods of no or minimal symptoms, the arterial P_{CO_2} is typically normal. With exacerbations, the P_{CO_2} may decrease to the middle or low 30s, possibly as a result of stimulation of the peripheral chemoreceptors by the mild hypoxemia or stimulation of intrapulmonary receptors. The P_{CO_2} is prevented from rising by increased ventilation to the alveoli in the face of the ventilation–perfusion inequality (compare Figure 2.10). In status asthmaticus, the arterial P_{CO_2} may rise while the pH falls. This is an ominous development that denotes impending respiratory failure and signals the need for urgent and intensive treatment, including possibly mechanical ventilatory support (see Chapter 10).

The diffusing capacity for carbon monoxide is typically normal or high in uncomplicated asthma. If it is reduced, associated emphysema should be suspected. The reason for the increased diffusing capacity is probably the large lung volume. Hyperinflation increases the diffusing capacity in normal subjects, presumably by increasing the area of the blood–gas interface.

Treatment of Patients with Asthma

Effective treatment of asthma relies on identification and elimination of triggers as well medications that address the underlying airway inflammation and reverse or prevent bronchoconstriction. These medications fall in two general classes, "controller" medications used on a regular basis to suppress airway inflammation and "reliever," or "rescue" medications used on an as-needed basis for acute symptoms.

Inhaled Corticosteroids

Because asthma is inherently an inflammatory disorder, inhaled corticosteroids are the primary controller medication (i.e., routine daily use) in all patients with persistent disease of any severity. This is in contrast to COPD, where inhaled corticosteroids are reserved for those with more severe disease. They appear to have two separate functions: inhibiting the inflammatory/immune response and enhancing β-receptor expression or function. Current guidelines recommend inhaled corticosteroids for patients with symptoms more than twice a week, inhaled β-agonist use more than twice a week, or frequent nighttime awakenings due to asthma symptoms. A wide variety of inhaled corticosteroids are now available and, when used as directed, result in minimal systemic absorption of corticosteroid with almost no serious side effects. In many cases, patients use combination inhalers that deliver both a corticosteroid and a β_2-agonist.

β-Adrenergic Agonists

β-Adrenergic receptors are of two types: β_1-receptors exist in the heart and elsewhere, and their stimulation increases heart rate and the force of contraction of cardiac muscle. Stimulation of β_2-receptors relaxes smooth muscle in the bronchi, blood vessels, and uterus. Partially or completely β_2-selective adrenergic agonists have now completely replaced nonselective agonists, with the most commonly used agents being albuterol and levalbuterol. These short-acting agents are typically used as reliever medications. Long-acting agents, such as formoterol and salmeterol, can be used as a controller but should always be used in combination with inhaled corticosteroids. All these drugs bind to β_2-receptors in the lung and directly relax airway smooth muscle by increasing the activity of adenyl cyclase. This, in turn, raises the concentration of intracellular cAMP, which is reduced in an asthma attack (Figure 4.14). They also have effects on airway edema and airway inflammation. Their anti-inflammatory effects are mediated by direct inhibition of inflammatory cell function via binding to β_2-receptors on the cell surface. There is some polymorphism in these receptors that affects the responses.

Medications Used for Asthma

Inhaled Corticosteroids
These are given by aerosol and are indicated except in the mildest cases of asthma.

β-Adrenergic Agonists
Selective β_2 types are now exclusively used.

Long-acting forms are useful in prolonged management, especially in conjunction with inhaled corticosteroids.

Short-acting forms are reserved for rescue.

Auxiliary Drugs
Antileukotrienes, antimuscarinics methylxanthine, cromolyn, and anti-IL5 or anti-IgE agents may be useful adjuncts.

Antimuscarinics

While antimuscarinics are used extensively in management of patients with COPD, they are generally not part of the treatment regimen in the majority of asthma patients. This is despite some evidence that the parasympathetic system plays a role in asthma pathophysiology. Some recent evidence suggests the long-acting antimuscarinic tiotropium may have benefit in patients with persistent symptoms despite intensive therapy with inhaled corticosteroids and β_2-agonists, but this is not presently standard practice.

Cromolyn and Nedocromil

Although their precise mechanism of action remains unclear, these two drugs are thought to prevent bronchoconstriction by stabilizing mast cells (Figure 4.15) and other broad ranging effects. Their use is generally limited to prophylaxis in situations known to provoke symptoms such as prior to exercise in cold, dry conditions or visiting an environment with a known trigger for the particular individual such as a home with a cat.

Methylxanthines
Methylxanthines, including theophylline and aminophylline inhibit phosphodiesterases in bronchial smooth muscle, leading to bronchodilation. While used more extensively in the past, they are used little in current practice because of modest anti-inflammatory and bronchodilatory activity relative to corticosteroids and β_2-agonists, risk for toxicity, and the need for monitoring serum concentrations on a regular basis.

Leukotriene-Modifying Drugs
Because leukotrienes C4, D4, and E4 mediate part of the allergic response in asthma, leukotriene receptor antagonists (e.g., montelukast, zafirlukast) and 5-lipoxygenase inhibitors (e.g., zileuton) are now used in some individuals. In well-selected patients with mild to moderate disease, they can be used in lieu of inhaled corticosteroids, while in more severe forms of disease, they may provide benefit when added to existing treatment with inhaled corticosteroids. They may be of particular use to patients whose asthma is exacerbated by aspirin and other nonsteroidal anti-inflammatory drugs.

Biologic Therapy
Several drugs are now available that target specific components of the inflammatory pathway of asthma. The monoclonal antibody to IgE, Omalizumab, can be used in patients with moderate to severe asthma who are inadequately controlled with high doses of inhaled glucocorticoids and have elevated serum IgE levels and evidence of allergen sensitization. Use has been limited by difficulties predicting which patients respond to therapy, the very high cost, and the risk of hypersensitivity reactions including anaphylaxis. Antibodies to IL-5 (mepolizumab and reslizumab) and antibodies to the IL-5 receptor (benralizumab) can also be used in selected patients with difficult to control disease.

General Approach to Treatment
Which medications are appropriate for a given patient depends on the adequacy of asthma control. Patients with sporadic symptoms typically only use reliever medications on an as-needed basis. While this has traditionally been a short-acting β_2-agonist, recent evidence suggests a combination corticosteroid β_2-agonist inhaler may be more effective at preventing exacerbations. Patients with persistent symptoms require a controller medication, typically an inhaled corticosteroid. Worsening asthma control is addressed by increasing the dose of the steroid and/or adding one or more of the other agents discussed above. Acute exacerbations are managed with a combination of systemically delivered corticosteroids and aggressive administration of inhaled

β$_2$-agonists. In very severe cases, intravenous magnesium or subcutaneous epinephrine may be used to promote bronchodilation. Mechanical ventilatory support may also be required.

LOCALIZED AIRWAY OBSTRUCTION

So far, this chapter has been devoted to generalized airway obstruction, both irreversible, as in emphysema and chronic bronchitis, and reversible, as in asthma. (Some chronic bronchitis may show some reversibility.) Localized obstruction is less common and associated with varying degrees of functional impairment depending on the nature and severity of the obstruction. Obstruction may be within the lumen of the airway, in the wall, or as a result of compression from outside the wall (Figure 4.1).

Tracheal Obstruction

This can be caused by an inhaled foreign body, stenosis after the use of an indwelling tracheotomy tube, intraluminal masses, or compression from extraluminal masses, such as an enlarged thyroid or massive mediastinal lymphadenopathy (Figure 4.19). There is inspiratory and expiratory stridor, abnormal inspiratory and expiratory flow–volume curves (see Figure 1.9), and no response to bronchodilators. Hypoventilation may result in hypercapnia and hypoxemia (see Figure 2.2).

Bronchial Obstruction

This is often caused by inhalation of a foreign body, such as a peanut or marble. The right lung is more frequently affected than the left because the left main bronchus makes a sharper angle with the trachea than does the right. Other common causes are malignant or benign bronchial tumors

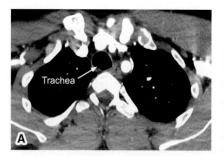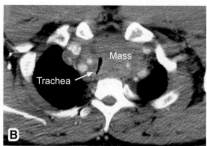

Figure 4.19. An example of upper airway obstruction. A. The *white arrow* points the normal diameter trachea in a healthy individual. **B.** The *white arrow* highlights a trachea that is markedly narrowed due to compression by a mass lesion located outside the airway. The mass was determined to be lymphadenopathy secondary to lymphoma.

and compression of a bronchus by enlarged surrounding lymph nodes. This last cause particularly affects the right middle lobe bronchus because of its anatomic relationships.

If obstruction is complete, absorption atelectasis occurs because the sum of the partial pressures in mixed venous blood is less than that in alveolar gas. (See *West's Respiratory Physiology: The Essentials*, 11th ed., p. 180.) The collapsed lobe is often visible on the radiograph, and compensatory overinflation of adjacent lung and displacement of a fissure may also be seen. Perfusion of the unventilated lung is reduced because of hypoxic pulmonary vasoconstriction and also the increased vascular resistance caused by the mechanical effects of the reduced volume on the extra-alveolar vessels and the capillaries. However, the residual blood flow contributes to hypoxemia. The most sensitive test is the alveolar–arterial P_{O_2} difference during 100% O_2 breathing (see Figure 2.6). Infection may follow localized obstruction and lead to lung abscess. If the obstruction is in a segmental or smaller bronchus, atelectasis may not occur because of collateral ventilation (see Figure 1.11). Long-standing unresolved bronchial obstruction can lead to infection and bronchiectasis distal to the obstruction.

KEY CONCEPTS

1. Chronic obstructive pulmonary disease is extremely common and can be very disabling. These patients have emphysema, chronic bronchitis, or a mixture of both.

2. Emphysema is a disease of the lung parenchyma characterized by the breakdown of alveolar walls with loss of lung elastic recoil and dynamic compression of airways.

3. Chronic bronchitis refers to inflammation of the airways with excessive mucus production. The lung parenchyma is normal or nearly so.

4. Asthma is characterized by increased responsiveness of the airways due to underlying inflammation. The airway narrowing typically varies in severity over time.

5. All of these diseases cause marked changes in forced expiration with reductions in the FEV_1, FVC, and FEV_1/FVC.

6. In addition to smoking cessation, inhaled β_2-adrenergic agonists and antimuscarinics are the mainstay of therapy for patients with COPD. Inhaled corticosteroids are usually reserved for severely affected patients.

7. Asthma can be treated effectively with inhaled corticosteroids and β_2-adrenergic agonists.

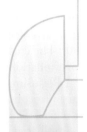

CLINICAL VIGNETTE

A 26-year-old man comes to the emergency department with worsening dyspnea and chest tightness over a 2-day period. He has had increasing nonproductive cough and states that he feels as if he can't get air into his chest on inhalation. He was diagnosed with asthma several years ago and has been treated with a daily inhaled corticosteroid and short-acting β_2-agonist, as needed, for several years with good improvement. However, following an upper respiratory tract infection that started several days ago, he has taken his β_2-agonist on a more frequent basis for relief of increased symptoms. Today, he has had little relief with the inhaler and decided to seek further help. On examination in the emergency department, his vital signs include temperature 37.0°C, heart rate 110, blood pressure 110/75, respiratory rate 25, and S_pO_2 92% breathing ambient air. His sternocleidomastoid and intercostal muscles are visibly contracting. He has diffuse, musical sounds through his bilateral lung fields and a prolonged expiratory phase. A chest radiograph shows no focal opacities but enlarged rib spaces and flattened diaphragms bilaterally.

Questions

- How would his functional residual capacity and residual volume at present compare to when he is in his normal healthy state?
- Why does he feel as if he cannot inhale adequately when asthma is a disease of airflow obstruction on exhalation?
- What is the most likely cause of his hypoxemia?
- If you were to obtain an arterial blood sample, what change would you expect to see in his arterial P_{CO_2}?
- What treatment is appropriate at this time?

QUESTIONS

For each question, choose the best answer.

1. A 29-year-old man presents to his primary care provider with increasing dyspnea and chest tightness. His symptoms, which are typically episodic and triggered by exercise, started worsening at the onset of spring a few weeks ago. They have markedly increased in the past 3 days, such that he is now using his albuterol inhaler multiple times per day, including several times at night. On exam, he is tachypneic and has diffuse end-expiratory wheezes and intercostal muscle retraction. If the patient underwent pulmonary function testing at this time, which of the following parameters would be increased compared to the predicted value?

A. FEF$_{25\%-75\%}$
B. FEV$_1$
C. FEV$_1$/FVC
D. Peak expiratory flow rate
E. Residual volume

2. After a fall down a staircase at home, a 71-year-old man with a several year history of exercise intolerance undergoes a CT scan of the chest in the emergency department. Two images from this scan are shown in the figure below.

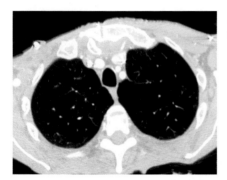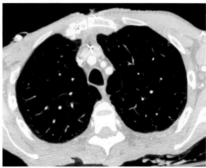

Which of the following is the most likely underlying cause of the changes in the lung parenchyma observed in the CT scan?
A. Bronchial smooth muscle hypertrophy and hyperplasia
B. Excess collagen deposition in the interstitial space
C. Excess release of neutrophil elastase and destruction of elastin
D. Infiltration of the airway walls by eosinophils and lymphocytes
E. Long-standing unresolved bronchial obstruction

3. The figure below displays the distribution of ventilation–perfusion ratios in two patients with chronic obstructive pulmonary disease.

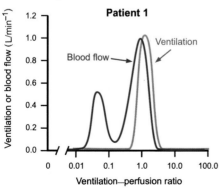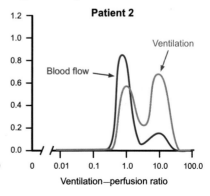

Which of these two patients is more likely to develop hypoxemia?
A. Patient 1
B. Patient 2

4. A 58-year-old man with a 60 pack-year history of smoking comes to the clinic because of worsening dyspnea over a 1-year period. He has no cough. On exam, he is a thin man with scattered musical sounds heard on auscultation and a prolonged expiratory phase. Spirometry performed in clinic shows an FEV_1 45% predicted, FVC 65% predicted, and FEV_1/FVC 0.58. Which of the following would most likely be seen in PA and lateral chest radiographs in this patient?
A. Bilateral hilar lymphadenopathy
B. Decreased size of the retrosternal airspace
C. Decreased vascular markings
D. Diffuse, bilateral lung opacities
E. Reticular opacities at the lung bases

5. A 22-year-old woman presents with episodic dyspnea, chest tightness, and cough. She was seen several months ago for these symptoms at an urgent care clinic and was given an albuterol inhaler, which provided symptomatic relief. She has been using it over five times per week and at least two times per week at night when she awakens with symptoms. Spirometry reveals an FEV_1 65% predicted, FVC 80% predicted, and FEV_1/FVC 0.65. All of these measurements improve significantly following administration of a short-acting bronchodilator. Which of the following medications is indicated for daily use for improved disease control?
A. Anti-IgE therapy
B. Cromolyn
C. Inhaled corticosteroid
D. Inhaled long-acting antimuscarinic
E. Inhaled long-acting β_2-agonist

6. A 38-year-old man with a 10 pack-year history of smoking presents to the pulmonary clinic for evaluation of worsening dyspnea on exertion. He has an intermittent cough but denies sputum production. On exam, he lacks stridor but has bilateral, diffuse expiratory wheezes and a long expiratory phase. Pulmonary function testing reveals airflow obstruction without a bronchodilator response. A plain chest radiograph demonstrates large lung volumes, flat diaphragms, and increased lucency in the bilateral lower lung zones, while an abdominal ultrasound shows evidence of a small, nodular liver. Which of the following is the most likely problem in this patient?

A. Asthma
B. Centriacinar emphysema
C. Chronic bronchitis
D. Obstructing tumor of the trachea
E. Panacinar emphysema

7. A 63-year-old woman is evaluated for worsening dyspnea on exertion over an 18-month period. She is a retired teacher with a 30-year history of smoking. Her spirometry reveals an FEV_1 59% predicted, FVC 78% predicted, and FEV_1/FVC ratio 0.62 with no response to inhaled bronchodilators. A chest radiograph demonstrates large lung volumes, a large retrosternal airspace, and flattened diaphragms. Which of the following would most likely be seen on further pulmonary function testing in this patient?
   A. Decreased functional residual capacity
   B. Decreased residual volume
   C. Decreased total lung capacity
   D. Increased diffusing capacity for carbon monoxide
   E. Increased RV/TLC ratio

8. A 16-year-old girl with a history of asthma is brought into the emergency department with chest tightness and wheezing that have not improved despite using her inhaled bronchodilator. On exam, she has an oxygen saturation of 92% breathing ambient air and use of accessory muscles of respiration and diffuse musical sounds on expiration. An arterial blood gas is drawn and shows a P_{CO_2} 33 mm Hg and P_{O_2} 59 mm Hg. The P_{O_2} improves to 90 mm Hg with administration of 2 L/min of oxygen by nasal cannula. Which of the following is the most likely cause of her hypoxemia?
   A. Diffusion impairment
   B. Hyperventilation
   C. Hypoventilation
   D. Shunt
   E. Ventilation–perfusion mismatch

9. A 34-year-old woman presents for evaluation of dyspnea and wheezing that has worsened over a several month period. She lives with a friend and her two cats and notes ongoing problems with mold in their old apartment. She has smoked one-half pack of cigarettes per day for 15 years. Pulmonary function testing is performed and reveals an FEV_1 2.51 liters (81% predicted), FVC 3.66 liters (92% predicted), and an FEV_1/FVC of 0.69. There is no significant improvement with bronchodilators. The flow volume loop is displayed in the figure below.

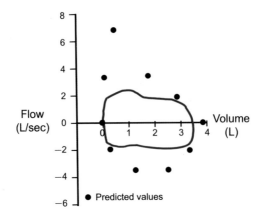

Which of the following is the most appropriate next step in the evaluation and management of this patient?

A. Measure the diffusion capacity for carbon monoxide.
B. Refer for bronchoscopy for airway inspection.
C. Refer for a cardiopulmonary exercise test.
D. Start a long-acting inhaled beta-agonist.
E. Start an inhaled corticosteroid.

10. While working in the pulmonary function laboratory, you are reviewing studies performed on a patient with asthma whose symptoms have been much more active lately and a patient with emphysema. The technologist forgot to label the results with the patients' names and you are trying to determine which results belong to which patient. The data from the tests are shown in the table below.

Test	Patient 1	Patient 2
FEV_1	75% predicted	71% predicted
FVC	78% predicted	77% predicted
FEV_1/FVC	0.65	0.59
RV	119% predicted	123% predicted
D_LCO	82% predicted	45% predicted

Which of the two patients is the one with emphysema?

A. Patient 1
B. Patient 2

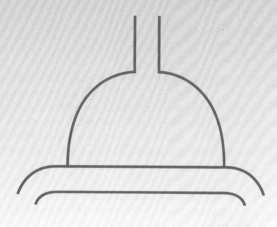

Restrictive Diseases

5

Restrictive diseases are those in which the expansion of the lung is restricted either because of alterations in the lung parenchyma or because of extraparenchymal disease involving the pleura, chest wall, or neuromuscular apparatus. They are characterized by a reduced vital capacity and a small resting lung volume (usually), but the airway resistance (related to lung volume) is not increased. These diseases are therefore different from the obstructive diseases in their pure form, although mixed restrictive and obstructive conditions can occur. At the end of this chapter, the reader should be able to:

- Describe the pathological and clinical features of idiopathic pulmonary fibrosis
- Identify the cause of hypoxemia and other key changes in pulmonary function in idiopathic pulmonary fibrosis
- Use clinical data to identify patients with sarcoidosis and hypersensitivity pneumonitis
- Describe the causes and general approach to evaluation and management of pneumothoraces and pleural effusions
- Distinguish between parenchymal and extraparenchymal causes of lung restriction on pulmonary function testing

DISEASES OF THE LUNG PARENCHYMA

This term refers to the alveolar tissue of the lung. A brief review of the structure of this tissue is pertinent.

Structure of the Alveolar Wall

Figure 5.1 shows an electron micrograph of a pulmonary capillary in an alveolar wall. The various structures through which oxygen passes on its way from the alveolar gas to the hemoglobin of the red blood cell are the layer of pulmonary surfactant (not shown in this preparation), alveolar epithelium, interstitium, capillary endothelium, plasma, and erythrocyte.

Cell Types

The various cell types have different functions and different responses to injury.

Type 1 Epithelial Cell This is the chief structural cell of the alveolar wall; its long cytoplasmic extensions pave almost the whole alveolar surface (Figure 5.1). The main function of this cell is mechanical support. It rarely divides and is not very active metabolically. When type 1 cells are injured, they are replaced by type 2 cells, which later transform into type 1 cells.

Type 2 Epithelial Cell This is a nearly globular cell (Figure 5.2) that gives little structural support to the alveolar wall but is metabolically active. The electron micrograph shows the lamellated bodies that contain phospholipids.

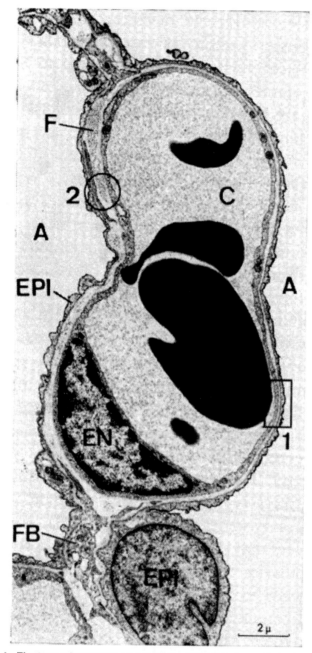

Figure 5.1. Electron micrograph of a portion of an alveolar wall. A, alveolar
space; EPI, type I alveolar epithelial cell nucleus and cytoplasm; C, capillary lumen;
EN, endothelial cell nucleus; FB, fibroblast; F, collagen fibrils; 1, thin region of blood–gas
barrier; 2, thick region of blood–gas barrier. (Reprinted from Weibel ER. Morphological
basis of alveolar-capillary gas exchange. Physiol Res. 1973;53(2):419-495. Copyright ©
1973 by American *Physiological Society*. All rights reserved.)

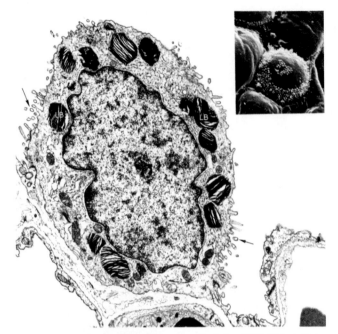

Figure 5.2. **Electron micrograph of type 2 epithelial cell (10,000×).** Note the lamellated bodies (*LB*), large nucleus, and microvilli (*arrows*), which are mainly concentrated around the edge of the cell, and cytoplasm rich in organelles. The inset at top right is a scanning electron micrograph showing the surface view of a type 2 cell with its characteristic distribution of microvilli (3,400×). (Republished with permission of Springer, from Weibel ER, Gil J. Structure–function relationships at the alveolar level. In: West JB. ed. *Bioengineering Aspects of the Lung.* New York, NY: Marcel Dekker; 1977; permission conveyed through Copyright Clearance Center, Inc.)

This is formed in the endoplasmic reticulum, passed through the Golgi apparatus, and eventually extruded into the alveolar space to form surfactant. (See *West's Respiratory Physiology: The Essentials*, 11th ed., p. 122-123.) After injury to the alveolar wall, these cells rapidly divide to line the surface and then later transform into type 1 cells. A type 3 cell has also been described, but it is rare and its function is unknown.

Alveolar Macrophage This scavenger cell roams around the alveolar wall phagocytosing foreign particles and bacteria. The cell contains lysozymes that digest engulfed foreign matter.

Fibroblast This cell synthesizes collagen and elastin, which are components of the interstitium of the alveolar wall. After various disease insults, large amounts of these materials may be laid down. This results in interstitial fibrosis.

Interstitium

This fills the space between the alveolar epithelium and the capillary endothelium. Figure 5.1 shows that it is thin on one side of the capillary, where it consists only of the fused basement membranes of the epithelial and endothelial layers. On the other side of the capillary, the interstitium is usually wider and includes fibrils of type I collagen. The thick side is chiefly concerned with fluid exchange across the endothelium, whereas the thin side is responsible for most of the gas exchange.

Interstitial tissue is found elsewhere in the lung, notably in the perivascular and peribronchial spaces around the larger blood vessels and airways and in the interlobular septa. The interstitium of the alveolar wall is continuous with that in the perivascular spaces (see Figure 6.1) and is the route by which fluid drains from the capillaries to the lymphatics.

Idiopathic Pulmonary Fibrosis

This is a form of diffuse interstitial fibrosis that develops in the absence of a clear precipitating factor. Historically, the nomenclature of this condition has been confusing, with many terms used in reference to it, including interstitial pneumonia, and cryptogenic fibrosing alveolitis. Diffuse fibrosis is the end stage of many diseases affecting the lung parenchyma. As a result, the changes in pulmonary function described in detail below are typical of advanced forms of many of the other parenchymal diseases alluded to later in this chapter.

Pathology

The histopathologic equivalent of idiopathic pulmonary fibrosis (IPF) is referred to as usual interstitial pneumonia (UIP). The principal feature is thickening of the interstitium of the alveolar wall. Initially, there is infiltration with lymphocytes and plasma cells (see Figure 2.5). Later, fibroblasts appear and lay down thick collagen bundles (Figure 5.3). These changes may be dispersed irregularly within the lung. In some patients, a cellular exudate consisting of macrophages and other mononuclear cells is seen within the alveoli in the early stages of the disease. This is called "desquamation." Eventually, the alveolar architecture is destroyed and the scarring results in multiple air-filled cystic spaces formed by dilated terminal and respiratory bronchioles, so-called honeycomb lung.

Pathogenesis

This is unknown, although in some cases there is evidence of an immunologic reaction.

Clinical Features

The disease is not common and tends to affect adults in the fifth to seventh decades of life. The patient often presents with dyspnea, that is typically more significant on exercise, as well as rapid, shallow breathing. Patients often have

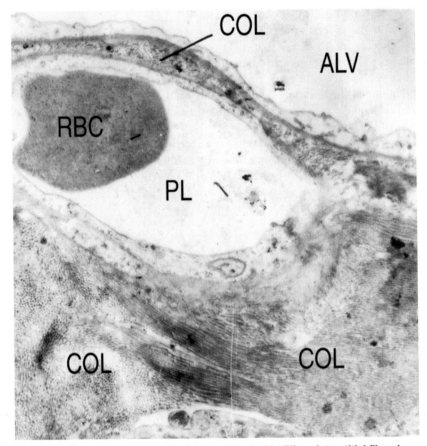

Figure 5.3. Electron micrograph from a patient with diffuse interstitial fibrosis.
Note the thick bundles of collagen. COL, collagen; ALV, alveolar space; RBC, red blood
cell; PL, plasma. Compare Figure 5.1. (Reprinted from Gracey DR, Divertie MD, Brown
AL Jr. Alveolar–capillary membrane in idiopathic interstitial pulmonary fibrosis. Electron
microscopic study of 14 cases. *Am Rev Respir Dis.* 1968;98(1):16–21. Copyright © 1968
American Thoracic Society. All Rights Reserved.)

an irritating, unproductive cough but lack fevers, hemoptysis, chest pain, and
constitutional symptoms.

On examination, mild cyanosis may be seen at rest in severe cases. It typically worsens on exercise. Fine crepitations, often referred to as crackles, are
usually heard throughout both lungs, especially toward the end of inspiration. Finger clubbing is common. The chest radiograph (Figure 5.4) shows
small lung volumes and a reticular (i.e., net-like) or reticulonodular pattern,
especially at the bases. Patchy shadows near the diaphragm may be caused by
basal collapse. Late in the disease, a honeycomb pattern develops, which is
best appreciated on a CT scan of the chest; this is caused by multiple airspaces
surrounded by thickened tissue (Figure 5.5) and is often most prominent in

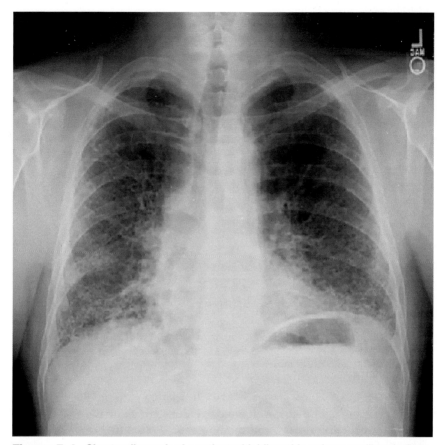

Figure 5.4. Chest radiograph of a patient with idiopathic pulmonary fibrosis. Note the small contracted lung and ribcage and the raised diaphragms. Net-like or "reticular" opacities are present in both lungs, particularly at the lung bases. Compare the normal appearance in Figure 4.8A.

the bases and periphery of the lung. CT may also show airways that are pulled open by surrounding fibrous tissue, a phenomenon referred to as traction dilatation or traction bronchiectasis.

Cor pulmonale may develop as a complication of advanced disease. The diseases often progress insidiously and patients typically die from progressive respiratory failure. Some patients develop acute exacerbations over a period of days to weeks that are associated with a very high risk of mortality.

Pulmonary Function

Ventilatory Capacity and Mechanics Spirometry typically reveals a restrictive pattern (see Figure 1.2). The FVC is markedly reduced, but the gas is exhaled rapidly so that although the FEV_1 is low, the FEV_1/FVC ratio is normal or is abnormally high. The almost square shape of the forced expiratory

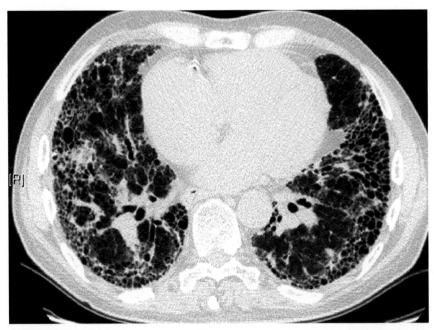

Figure 5.5. Single slice of a chest CT scan of a patient with idiopathic pulmonary fibrosis. Note the extensive septal thickening and the prominent honeycombing, particularly in the periphery of the lungs.

spirogram is in striking contrast to the obstructive pattern. The $FEF_{25-75\%}$ is normal or high. The flow–volume curve does not show the scooped-out shape of obstructive disease, and the flow rate is often higher than normal when related to absolute lung volume. This is shown in Figure 1.5, where it can be seen that the downslope of the curve for restrictive disease lies above the normal curve.

All lung volumes are reduced, including the TLC, FRC, and RV, but the relative proportions are more or less preserved. The pressure–volume curve of the lung is flattened and displaced downward (see Figure 3.1), so that at any given volume, the transpulmonary pressure is abnormally high. The maximum elastic recoil pressure that can be generated at TLC is typically higher than normal.

All these results are consistent with the pathologic appearance of fibrosis of the alveolar walls (Figures 2.5 and 5.3). The fibrous tissue reduces the distensibility of the lung just as a scar on the skin reduces its distensibility. As a result, the lung volumes are small, and abnormally large pressures are required to distend the lung. The airways may not be specifically involved, but they tend to narrow as lung volume is reduced. However, airway resistance at a given lung volume is normal or even decreased because the retractile forces exerted on the airway walls by the surrounding parenchyma are abnormally high (Figure 5.5). The pathologic correlate of this is the honeycomb appearance caused by the dilated terminal and respiratory bronchioles surrounded by thickened scar tissue.

Gas Exchange The arterial P_{O_2} and P_{CO_2} are typically reduced, and the pH is normal. The hypoxemia is usually mild at rest until the disease is advanced. However, on exercise, the P_{O_2} often falls dramatically. In well-established disease, both the physiologic dead space and the physiologic shunt are increased.

The relative contribution of diffusion impairment and ventilation–perfusion ($\dot{V}_A/\dot{Q}$) inequality to the hypoxemia of these patients has long been debated. It is natural to argue that the histologic appearances shown in Figures 2.5 and 5.3 slow the diffusion of oxygen from the alveolar gas to the capillary blood because the thickness of the barrier may be increased many fold (compare Figure 2.5 with Figure 5.1). In addition, the increasing hypoxemia during exercise is consistent with the mechanism of impaired diffusion because exercise reduces the time spent by the red cells in the pulmonary capillary (Figure 2.4).

Features of Pulmonary Function in Idiopathic Pulmonary Fibrosis

- Dyspnea with shallow, rapid breathing
- Reductions in all lung volumes
- FEV_1/FVC ratio normal or even increased
- Airway resistance normal or low when related to lung volume
- Reduced lung compliance
- Very negative intrapleural pressure at TLC
- Arterial hypoxemia chiefly due to $\dot{V}_A/\dot{Q}$ inequality
- Diffusion impairment possibly contributing to the hypoxemia during exercise
- Normal or low arterial P_{CO_2}
- Reduced diffusing capacity for carbon monoxide
- Increased pulmonary vascular resistance

However, we now know that impaired diffusion is not the chief cause of the hypoxemia in these conditions. First, the normal lung has enormous reserves of diffusion in that the P_{O_2} of the blood nearly reaches that in alveolar gas early in its transit through the capillary (see Figure 2.4). In addition, these patients have substantial inequality of ventilation and blood flow within the lung, as demonstrated by single-breath nitrogen washouts and measurements of topographical function with radioactive gases. How could they not, with the disorganization of architecture shown in Figures 2.5 and 5.3?

To apportion blame for the hypoxemia between the two possible mechanisms, it is necessary to measure the degree of $\dot{V}_A/\dot{Q}$ inequality and determine

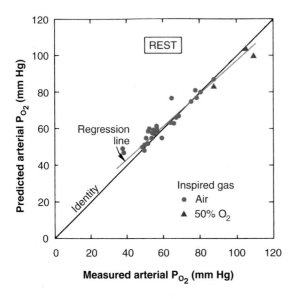

Figure 5.6. Study of the mechanism of hypoxemia in a series of patients with interstitial lung disease. This figure shows that the arterial P_{O_2} predicted from the pattern of $\dot{V}_A/\dot{Q}$ inequality agreed well with the measured arterial P_{O_2}. Thus, at rest, all of the hypoxemia could be explained by the uneven ventilation and blood flow.

how much of the hypoxemia is attributable to this. This has been done by using the multiple inert gas elimination technique in a series of patients with interstitial lung disease. Figure 5.6 shows that at rest, the hypoxemia could be adequately explained by the degree of $\dot{V}_A/\dot{Q}$ inequality in these patients. However, Figure 5.7 shows that on exercise, the observed alveolar P_{O_2} was generally below the value predicted from the measured amount of $\dot{V}_A/\dot{Q}$ inequality, and thus, an additional cause of hypoxemia must have been present. Most likely, this was diffusion impairment in these patients. Importantly, hypoxemia

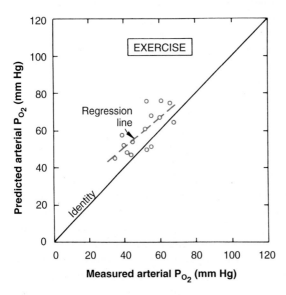

Figure 5.7. Results obtained on exercise in the same patients as shown in Figure 5.6. Under these conditions, the measured arterial P_{O_2} was below that predicted from the pattern of $\dot{V}_A/\dot{Q}$ inequality. This indicates an additional mechanism for hypoxemia, presumably diffusion impairment.

caused by diffusion impairment was evident only on exercise, and even then, it accounted for only about one-third of the alveolar–arterial P_{O_2} difference.

The low arterial P_{CO_2} in these patients (typically in the low to middle 30s) occurs despite the evident $\dot{V}_A/\dot{Q}$ inequality and is caused by increased ventilation to the alveoli (compare Figure 2.10). The cause of the increased ventilation is uncertain. There is some evidence that the control of ventilation is abnormal because of the stimulation of receptors within the lung (see later text). Stimulation of the peripheral chemoreceptors by the arterial hypoxemia may also be a factor. The arterial pH is usually normal at rest but may increase considerably on exercise as a result of the hyperventilation and consequent respiratory alkalosis (compare Figure 3.3), although metabolic acidosis caused by lactic acid accumulation may also occur in late exercise. In very advanced stages of IPF, severe abnormalities in lung mechanics can lead to hypoventilation with subsequent increases P_{CO_2}.

The diffusing capacity for carbon monoxide is often strikingly reduced in these patients to the neighborhood of 5 mL/min/mm Hg (normal value 25 to 30 depending on age and stature). In fact, the low diffusing capacity is a useful way to distinguish between parenchymal and extraparenchymal causes of restriction. Reduced values are seen with parenchymal causes of restriction, whereas extraparenchymal causes are associated with normal or only mildly reduced diffusing capacity. The reductions seen in parenchymal causes are due, in part, to thickening of the blood–gas barrier (Figure 2.5). Other factors that contribute to the low diffusing capacity in IPF include reductions in the blood volume of the pulmonary capillaries because many of the vessels are obliterated by the fibrotic process as well as $\dot{V}_A/\dot{Q}$ inequality, which causes uneven emptying of the lung. This highlights how the diffusing capacity should not be taken to reflect only the properties of the blood–gas barrier.

Exercise Patients with pulmonary fibrosis may show much more evidence of impaired pulmonary function on exercise than at rest. In many cases, the increase in ventilation and respiratory rate on exercise is greatly exaggerated. As a result of the high ventilation, which is out of proportion to the increase in O_2 uptake and CO_2 output, the alveolar and arterial P_{CO_2} fall and the alveolar P_{O_2} increases. However, as noted earlier, the arterial P_{O_2} falls, thus increasing the alveolar–arterial P_{O_2} difference. This result can be explained partly by the impaired diffusion characteristics of the lung (Figure 5.6). However, most of the hypoxemia on exercise is caused by $\dot{V}_A/\dot{Q}$ inequality.

One contributor to the $\dot{V}_A/\dot{Q}$ inequality is an abnormally small rise in cardiac output. This occurs because these patients typically have increased pulmonary vascular resistance due to obliteration of pulmonary capillaries by the interstitial fibrosis (see Figure 2.5) and hypertrophy of vascular smooth muscle and consequent narrowing of the small arteries. The high resistance and limited ability to recruit and distend the pulmonary vasculature leads to substantial increases in pulmonary artery pressure with exercise and, as a result, impaired cardiac function. If cardiac output does not rise sufficiently to meet the increased metabolic demand of exercising muscles, mixed venous P_{O_2} decreases (see Chapter 9). In the setting of $\dot{V}_A/\dot{Q}$ inequality, this worsens arterial oxygenation.

The importance of this factor can be seen if we consider some results obtained in the laboratory in a patient with interstitial lung disease. During exercise that raised the O_2 uptake from about 300 to 700 mL/min, the arterial P_{O_2} fell from 50 to 35 mm Hg. The rise in cardiac output was only from 4.6 to 5.7 L/min; the normal value for this level of exercise is approximately 10 L/min. As a result, the P_{O_2} in the mixed venous blood fell to 17 mm Hg (normal value is approximately 35 mm Hg). Calculations show that if the cardiac output had increased to 10 L/min and the pattern of $\dot{V}_A/\dot{Q}$ inequality remained unchanged, the arterial P_{O_2} would have been some 10 mm Hg higher.

If the diffusing capacity for carbon monoxide is measured in these patients during exercise, it typically remains low, whereas it may double or triple in healthy individuals.

Control of Ventilation We have already seen that these patients typically have shallow rapid breathing, especially on exercise. The reason for this is not certain, but it is possible that the pattern is caused by reflexes originating in pulmonary irritant receptors or J (juxtacapillary) receptors. The former lie in the bronchi or in the epithelial lining and may be stimulated by the increased traction on the airways caused by the increased elastic recoil of the lung (Figure 5.8). The J receptors are in the alveolar walls and could be stimulated by the fibrotic changes in the interstitium. No direct evidence of increased activity of either receptor is yet available in humans, but work in experimental animals suggests that these reflexes could cause rapid shallow breathing.

The rapid shallow pattern of breathing reduces the respiratory work in patients with reduced lung compliance. However, it also increases ventilation of the anatomic dead space at the expense of the alveoli, so a compromise must be reached.

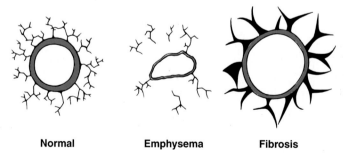

Normal   **Emphysema**   **Fibrosis**

Figure 5.8. Airway caliber in emphysema and interstitial fibrosis. In emphysema, the airways tend to collapse because of the loss of radial traction. By contrast, in fibrosis, radial traction may be excessive, with the result that airway caliber is large when related to lung volume.

Treatment and Outcomes

IPF is an invariably fatal process with the majority of people dying within 5 years of diagnosis. No treatment has been shown to improve mortality although the tyrosine kinase inhibitor nintedanib and the antifibrotic agent pirfenidone may slow the rate of decline in lung function and are now increasingly used in these patients. Lung transplantation is often pursued in patients who meet strict eligibility criteria.

Other Types of Parenchymal Restrictive Disease

The changes in pulmonary function in IPF have been dealt with at some length because this disease serves as an example of advanced forms of other parenchymal restrictive diseases. These diseases are now considered briefly here, and differences in their pattern of pulmonary function are discussed.

Sarcoidosis

This disease is characterized by the presence of granulomatous tissue having a characteristic histologic appearance. It often occurs in several organs.

Pathology The characteristic lesion is a noncaseating epithelioid granuloma composed of large histiocytes with giant cells and lymphocytes, which can occur in the lymph nodes, lungs, skin, eyes, liver, spleen, and elsewhere. In advanced pulmonary disease, fibrotic changes in the alveolar walls are seen.

Pathogenesis This is unknown, although an immunologic basis appears likely. One possibility is that an unknown antigen is recognized by an alveolar macrophage, which results in the activation of a T lymphocyte and the production of interleukin-2. The activated macrophage may also release various products that stimulate fibroblasts, thus explaining the deposition of fibrous tissue in the interstitium.

Clinical Features The clinical presentation of sarcoidosis varies from asymptomatic changes noted on chest radiography to severe multiorgan disease. Common pulmonary symptoms include dyspnea and dry cough, while extrapulmonary manifestations include arthritis, anterior uveitis, hypercalcemia, parotid gland enlargement, peripheral and central nervous system changes, and cardiac involvement such as conduction delays and restrictive cardiomyopathy.

Multiple stages of sarcoidosis can be identified based on the radiographic findings.

- *Stage 0*: There are no findings on plain chest radiography, although a CT scan may show enlarged mediastinal lymph nodes (lymphadenopathy).

- *Stage 1:* There is bilateral hilar adenopathy often with right paratracheal adenopathy (Figure 5.9). There are no disturbances of pulmonary function. When accompanied by polyarthralgias and erythema nodosum, this is referred to as Löfgren's syndrome.
- *Stage 2:* There is bilateral hilar adenopathy as well as reticular opacities, most significant in the mid and upper zones.
- *Stage 3:* There are reticular opacities in the mid-upper lung zones and shrinking hilar adenopathy.
- *Stage 4:* There is fibrosis, predominantly in the upper lobes. Low lung volumes and traction dilatation are often seen.

Even though multiple stages of the disease are described, patients do not necessarily progress from lower to higher stages. Many patients with lower stage disease are asymptomatic and are only identified as having sarcoidosis when radiographs are performed for other reasons (e.g., employment screening).

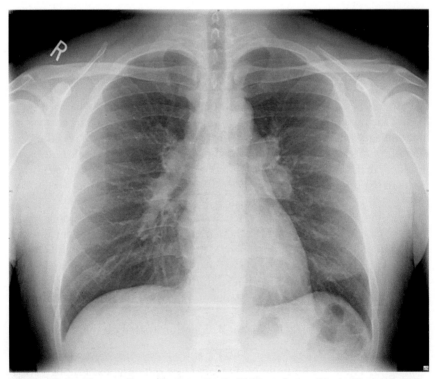

Figure 5.9. Chest radiograph of a patient with stage I sarcoidosis. The radiograph demonstrates bilateral hilar and right paratracheal lymphadenopathy but no parenchymal opacities.

Pulmonary Function There is no impairment of function in stages 0 and 1 of the disease. In stages 2 and 3, typical changes of the restrictive type are seen, although the radiographic appearance sometimes suggests more interference with function than actually exists.

Significant pulmonary fibrosis may develop in some patients, with a severe restrictive pattern of function. All lung volumes are small, but the FEV_1/FVC ratio is preserved. Lung compliance is strikingly reduced, the pressure–volume curve being flattened and shifted downward and to the right (see Figure 3.1). The resting arterial P_{O_2} is low and often falls considerably on exercise. The arterial P_{CO_2} is normal or low, although it may rise in severe disease as respiratory failure supervenes. The diffusing capacity for carbon monoxide (transfer factor) is reduced significantly. Cor pulmonale may develop in advanced disease.

Treatment Many patients with lower stage disease, including those with Löfgren's syndrome, require no treatment and experience spontaneous remission. Treatment, usually with systemic corticosteroids, is initiated in patients with worsening pulmonary function and increasing symptoms or extrapulmonary involvement.

Hypersensitivity Pneumonitis

Also referred to as extrinsic allergic alveolitis, hypersensitivity pneumonitis is a parenchymal lung disease that develops as a result of a type 3 (and occasionally Type 4) hypersensitivity reaction to inhaled organic dusts. The exposure is usually occupational and heavy but can occur in response to antigens in the home. Precipitins can be demonstrated in the serum.

The term "extrinsic" implies that the etiologic agent is external and can be identified, in contrast to "intrinsic" fibrosing alveolitis (idiopathic pulmonary fibrosis discussed above), where the cause is unknown. A very large number of exposures have been shown to cause hypersensitivity pneumonitis. Common examples include farmer's lung due to the spores of thermophilic *Actinomyces* in moldy hay, bird breeder's lung caused by avian antigens from feathers and excreta as well as air conditioner's lung and bagassosis (in sugarcane workers).

Pathology The alveolar walls are thickened and infiltrated with lymphocytes, plasma cells, and occasional eosinophils together with collections of histiocytes that, in some areas, form small granulomas that are less well organized than those seen in sarcoidosis. The small bronchioles are usually affected, and there may be exudate in the lumen. Fibrotic changes occur in advanced cases when exposure to the offending antigen persists for long periods of time.

Clinical Features The disease occurs in either acute or chronic forms. In the former, symptoms of dyspnea, fever, shivering, and cough appear 4 to 6 hours after exposure and continue for 24 to 48 hours. The patient is frequently dyspneic at rest, with fine crepitations throughout both lung fields. The disease may also occur in a chronic form without prior acute attacks. These patients present with progressive dyspnea, usually over a period of years. In the acute form, the chest radiograph may be normal, but frequently CT scans of the chest demonstrate a miliary nodular infiltrate or ground glass opacities. In the chronic form, fibrosis of the upper lobes is common and seen on both plain chest radiography and CT scans.

Pulmonary Function In well-developed disease, the typical restrictive pattern is seen. This includes reduced lung volumes, low compliance, hypoxemia that worsens on exercise, normal or low arterial P_{CO_2}, and a reduced diffusing capacity (Figure 3.3). In the early stages, variable degrees of airway obstruction may be present.

Treatment The most important treatment principle is elimination of the offending antigen. Some patients require long courses of systemic corticosteroids, but this may not lead to improvement if exposure to the offending antigen continues.

Interstitial Disease Caused by Drugs, Poisons, and Radiation

Various drugs may cause an acute pulmonary reaction, which can proceed to interstitial fibrosis. These drugs include the antibiotic nitrofurantoin, the cardiac antiarrhythmic agent amiodarone, novel antineoplastic agents, such as the immune checkpoint inhibitor nivolumab, and traditional antineoplastic drugs such as busulfan and bleomycin. Oxygen in high concentrations following bleomycin administration can cause acute toxic changes with subsequent interstitial fibrosis, even years after the patient received the medication (see Figure 5.3). Ingestion of the weed killer paraquat results in the rapid development of lethal interstitial fibrosis. Therapeutic radiation causes acute pneumonitis followed by fibrosis if lung is included in the field.

Asbestosis

Chronic exposure to asbestos fibers can lead to development of pulmonary fibrosis many years after the exposure. This entity, whose clinical features, pulmonary function, and gas exchange abnormalities resemble IPF, is described further in Chapter 7.

Collagen Vascular Diseases

Pulmonary fibrosis with a typical restrictive pattern may be found in patients with systemic sclerosis (generalized scleroderma). Dyspnea is often severe and out of proportion to the changes in radiologic appearance or lung function. Other connective tissue diseases that may produce fibrosis include systemic lupus erythematosus and rheumatoid arthritis.

Lymphangitis Carcinomatosis

This refers to the spread of carcinoma tissue through pulmonary lymphatics and may complicate carcinomas, chiefly of the breast, esophagus, lung, and stomach. Dyspnea is prominent, and the typical restrictive pattern of lung function may be seen.

DISEASES OF THE PLEURA

Pneumothorax

Air can enter the pleural space either from the lung or, less commonly, through the chest wall as a result of a penetrating wound. The pressure in the intrapleural space is normally subatmospheric as a result of the elastic recoil forces of the lung and chest wall. When air enters the space, intrapleural pressure increases, the lung collapses, and the rib cage springs out. These changes are evident on a chest radiograph (Figure 5.10), which shows partial or complete collapse of the lung, overexpansion of the rib cage, and depression of the diaphragm on the affected side, and sometimes displacement of the mediastinum away from the pneumothorax. These changes are most evident if the pneumothorax is large, particularly if a tension pneumothorax is present (see later text).

Spontaneous Pneumothorax

The causes of spontaneous pneumothorax are grouped into two categories. In *primary* spontaneous cases, pneumothorax develops without any predisposing lung disease. Typically occurring in tall young males, this form is caused by the rupture of a small bleb on the surface of the lung near the apex possibly due to the high mechanical stresses that occur in the upper zone of the upright lung (see Figure 3.3). In *secondary* spontaneous cases, the patient has an underlying lung disease such as COPD, cystic fibrosis, or pneumocystis pneumonia that predisposes to pneumothorax. It may also occur during mechanical ventilation with high airway pressures (see Chapter 10).

In either category, the presenting symptom is often sudden, unilateral pleuritic pain accompanied by dyspnea. On auscultation in patients with large pneumothoraces, breath sounds are reduced on the affected side. The diagnosis is readily confirmed by plain chest radiography. Identification of "lung sliding" on chest ultrasound can be used to confidently rule out the diagnosis.

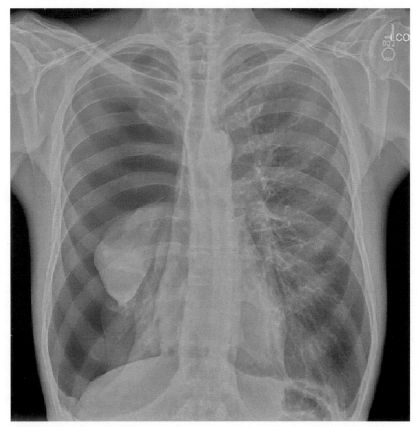

Figure 5.10. Chest radiograph showing a large right-sided spontaneous pneumothorax. Note the small, collapsed right lung.

If the hole in the lung seals over, the pneumothorax is gradually reabsorbed because the sum of the partial pressures in the venous blood is considerably less than atmospheric pressure. Tube thoracostomy may be necessary to resolve large pneumothoraces or in patients with underlying lung disease. This involves inserting a tube through the chest wall and connecting the tube to an underwater seal, allowing air to escape from the chest but not to enter it. Recurrent attacks may need surgical treatment to promote adhesions between the two pleural surfaces (pleurodesis).

Tension Pneumothorax

In a small proportion of pneumothoraces, the communication between the lung and the pleural space functions as a check valve. As a consequence, air enters the space during inspiration but cannot escape during expiration.

The result is a large pneumothorax in which the pressure may considerably exceed atmospheric pressure and thus interfere with venous return to the thorax.

This medical emergency is recognized by increasing respiratory distress, tachycardia, distended neck veins, and signs of mediastinal shift, such as tracheal deviation and displacement of the apex beat. While chest radiographs demonstrate characteristic changes including shift of the heart and mediastinal structures to the side opposite the pneumothorax, diagnosis should be made on clinical grounds before the radiograph is obtained. Treatment consists of urgently relieving the pressure by inserting a needle through the chest wall on the affected side then performing tube thoracostomy.

Spontaneous Pneumothorax

- Can occur in individuals with or without underlying lung diseases.
- Accompanied by sudden onset of dyspnea and pleuritic pain.
- Gradually absorbed by the blood.
- Tube thoracostomy may be required for large pneumothoraces.
- Recurrent attacks may require surgery.
- Tension pneumothorax is a medical emergency.

Pulmonary Function

As would be expected, a pneumothorax reduces the FEV_1 and FVC, but in practice, pulmonary function tests are rarely performed in the evaluation of acute dyspnea and would not be used in the diagnosis of pneumothorax.

Pleural Effusion

This refers to fluid rather than air in the pleural space. It is not a disease in its own right, but it frequently accompanies serious disease, and an explanation should always be sought. Pleural effusions typically develop as a result of imbalances in the Starling forces.

The patient often reports dyspnea if the effusion is large, and there may be pleuritic pain from the underlying disease. The chest signs are often informative and include reduced movement of the chest on the affected side, absence of breath sounds, and dullness to percussion. Chest radiographs, CT scans, and ultrasound can be used to identify pleural effusions (Figure 5.11A–C).

To diagnose the cause of an effusion, pleural fluid is sampled in a procedure called thoracentesis. Pleural effusions can be divided into exudates and transudates according to the results of pleural fluid analysis. Fluid is deemed exudative if the patient meets any one of three criteria: pleural fluid LDH

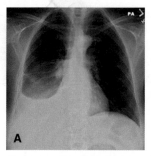 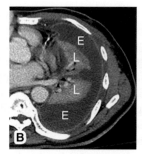 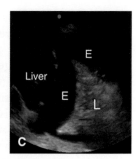

Figure 5.11. Appearance of pleural effusions on chest imaging. A. Plain chest radiograph. Note the dense, homogeneous opacity obscuring the right hemidiaphragm and right heart border. The upper margin of the opacity has a curvilinear appearance, referred to as a "meniscus sign," that his highly suggestive of effusion. **B.** Chest CT scan image. The lung (*L*) is compressed by the surrounding effusion (*E*). **C.** Ultrasound image showing an effusion (*E*), lung (*L*), and liver. The lung is more visible on ultrasound than normal because it is denser due to compression by the surrounding fluid. Note that the fluid is *black* on ultrasound, unlike on plain chest radiographs.

greater than two-third the upper limit of normal for the serum value, pleural fluid:serum LDH ratio greater than 0.6, or pleural fluid:serum protein ratio greater than 0.5. Recent data also suggest that pleural fluid cholesterol greater than 45 mg/dL is consistent with an exudate. Exudates can occur due to a large number of diseases but the most common causes are malignancies and infections. Transudates develop in severe heart failure, constrictive pericarditis, and other edematous states such as hypoalbuminemia, cirrhosis, and chronic kidney disease. While drainage of an effusion leads to symptomatic improvement, treatment should be directed at the underlying cause to prevent recurrence. Pulmonary function is impaired as in pneumothorax, but the measurements are not performed in practice.

Variants of pleural effusion include empyema (pyothorax), hemothorax, and chylothorax, which refer to the presence of pus, blood, and lymph, respectively, in the pleural space.

Pleural Thickening

Occasionally, a long-standing pleural effusion results in a rigid, contracted fibrotic pleura that splints the lung and prevents its expansion. This can result in a severe restrictive type of functional impairment, particularly if the disease is bilateral. Surgical stripping may be necessary.

DISEASES OF THE CHEST WALL

Kyphoscoliosis

Bony deformity of the chest can cause restrictive disease. "Scoliosis" refers to lateral curvature of the spine and kyphosis to posterior curvature. Scoliosis is more serious, especially if the angulation is high in the vertebral column. It is frequently associated with a backward protuberance of the ribs, giving the appearance of an added kyphosis. In most cases, the cause is unknown, although the condition can be caused by tuberculosis of the spine, neuromuscular disease, or repeated compression fractures of the spine with aging. The patient initially reports dyspnea on exertion; breathing tends to be rapid and shallow. Hypoxemia later develops, and eventually, carbon dioxide retention and cor pulmonale may supervene.

Pulmonary function tests typically show a reduction in all lung volumes. Airway resistance is nearly normal if related to lung volume. However, there is inequality of ventilation, partly because of airway closure in dependent regions. Parts of the lung are compressed, and there are often areas of atelectasis.

The hypoxemia is caused by ventilation–perfusion inequality. In advanced disease, a reduced ventilatory response to CO_2 can often be demonstrated. This reduction reflects the increased work of breathing caused by deformity of the chest wall. Not only is the chest wall stiff but also the respiratory muscles operate inefficiently. The pulmonary vascular bed is restricted, causing a rise in pulmonary artery pressure, which is exaggerated by the alveolar hypoxia. Venous congestion and peripheral edema may develop.

Ankylosing Spondylitis

In this inflammatory arthritis of the spine, there is a gradual but relentless onset of immobility of the vertebral joints and fixation of the ribs. As a result, the movement of the chest wall is grossly reduced. There is a reduction of FVC and TLC, but the FEV_1/FVC ratio and the airway resistance are normal. The compliance of the chest wall may fall, and there is often some uneven ventilation, probably secondary to the reduced lung volume. While the lung parenchyma remains normal in nearly all cases and diaphragmatic movement is preserved, a small percentage of patients develop fibrosis in the apical regions of the lungs.

NEUROMUSCULAR DISORDERS

Diseases affecting the muscles of respiration or their nerve supply include poliomyelitis, Guillain-Barré syndrome, amyotrophic lateral sclerosis, myasthenia gravis, botulism, and muscular dystrophies (see Table 2.1 and Figure 2.2). The inability of the patient to take in a deep breath is reflected in a reduced FEV_1, FVC, TLC, inspiratory capacity, and maximum inspiratory and expiratory pressures. The diffusing capacity for carbon monoxide is typically normal because the lung parenchyma is unaffected, although mild reductions are sometimes seen due to atelectasis at the base of the lungs.

Because the most important muscle of respiration is the diaphragm, patients with progressive neuromuscular disease often do not report dyspnea until the diaphragm is involved. The progress of the disease can be followed by monitoring changes in the FVC and arterial P_{CO_2} over time. By the time abnormalities are seen on these tests or patients are symptomatic, their ventilatory reserve may be severely compromised.

In rare cases, patients can develop isolated weakness of the diaphragm. This can be distinguished from diffuse neuromuscular disease by the fact that maximum inspiratory pressure is reduced while maximum expiratory pressure is preserved. Another hallmark of diaphragmatic weakness is a significant reduction in the FEV_1 and FVC when spirometry is repeated in the supine position. This finding can be seen in diffuse neuromuscular diseases as well.

KEY CONCEPTS

1. Idiopathic pulmonary fibrosis is an example of restrictive lung disease characterized by dyspnea, reduced exercise tolerance, small lungs, and reduced lung compliance.

2. In pulmonary fibrosis, the alveolar walls show marked infiltration with collagen and obliteration of capillaries.

3. Airway resistance is not increased in pulmonary fibrosis; indeed, a forced expiration can result in abnormally high flow rates because of the increased radial traction on the airway.

4. Diffusion of oxygen across the blood–gas barrier is impeded in pulmonary fibrosis by the thickening and may result in hypoxemia, especially on exercise. However, ventilation–perfusion inequality is the major factor in the impaired gas exchange at rest and with exercise.

5. Other restrictive disorders are caused by diseases of the pleura or chest wall or neuromuscular disease.

CLINICAL VIGNETTE

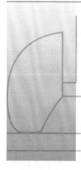

A 47-year-old woman is referred to the pulmonary clinic for evaluation of increasing dyspnea on exertion and fatigue. She is a dentist and is having increasing difficulty with her daily exercise in the gym. She has a chronic, nonproductive cough and denies hemoptysis, chest pain, fevers, arthralgias, rash, or ocular symptoms. On physical examination, her S_pO_2 is 93% breathing ambient air. She has end-inspiratory crackles in her bilateral lung fields, normal cardiac abdominal and skin exams, and no clubbing. A chest radiograph is obtained and reveals the following:

(Continued)

CLINICAL VIGNETTE (*Continued*)

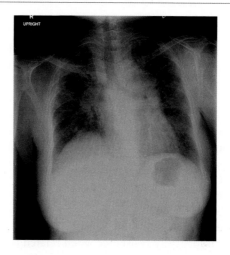

Parameter	Predicted	Prebron-chodilator	% Predicted	Postbron-chodilator	% Change
FVC (liters)	2.73	1.53	56	1.59	4
FEV$_1$ (liters)	2.28	1.12	49	1.10	-2
FEV$_1$/FVC	0.83	0.73	88	0.69	-6

Bronchoscopy is performed, and histopathologic examination of samples obtained via transbronchial biopsy reveals noncaseating granulomas.

Questions

- What changes would you expect to see in her TLC and diffusing capacity for carbon monoxide?
- How will her pressure–volume curve compare to that of a healthy individual?
- If you were to measure her arterial blood gases, what would you expect to find with her acid–base status?
- What will happen to her alveolar–arterial oxygen difference during exercise?

QUESTIONS

For each question, choose the one best answer.

1. A 67-year-old man, who is a life-long nonsmoker, complains of worsening dyspnea and dry cough over a 6-month period. On examination, he has a fast respiratory rate and is taking small breaths. He has fine crackles (crepitations) in the lower lung zones on auscultation and finger clubbing. A chest radiograph shows low lung volumes and reticulonodular opacities in the bilateral lower lung fields. Which of the following results would you expect to see on pulmonary function testing in this patient?
   A. Increased FEV_1
   B. Increased FVC
   C. Increased FEV_1/FVC
   D. Increased TLC
   E. Increased airway resistance when related to lung volume

2. A 52-year-old woman presents for evaluation of worsening dyspnea on exertion. A plain chest radiograph was obtained and demonstrated a right pleural effusion after which thoracentesis was performed. The results of her pleural fluid analysis are shown in the table below.

Test	Result
Pleural fluid protein	3.6 g/dL
Pleural fluid LDH	790 units/L
Pleural fluid cholesterol	75 mg/dL
Serum total protein	5.2 g/dL
Serum LDH	305 units/L

Which of the following is the most likely cause of her pleural effusion?
   A. Chronic kidney disease
   B. Cirrhosis
   C. Constrictive pericarditis
   D. Metastatic lung cancer
   E. Valvular cardiomyopathy

3. A 59-year-old man presents for evaluation of a 1-year history of progressive exercise intolerance and persistent dry cough. He has a 15 pack-year history of smoking, lives in the suburbs of a large city, works as an attorney, and has no birds or other pets at home. On examination, he has bilateral end-inspiratory crackles heard best at

the lung bases. Spirometry reveals an FEV_1 of 65% predicted, FVC 69% predicted, FEV_1/FVC 0.82, TLC 75% predicted, and diffusion capacity for carbon monoxide 53% predicted. His plain chest radiograph and a slice from his CT scan are shown in the figure below.

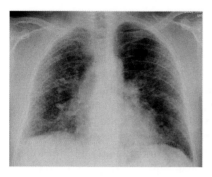 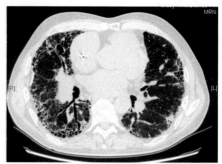

Which of the following would you expect on histopathologic examination of a lung biopsy specimen in this patient?
A. Caseating granulomas
B. Chronic inflammation and hypertrophied mucous glands
C. Enlarged airspaces with loss of alveolar walls
D. Smooth muscle hypertrophy
E. Thickened alveolar walls with increased collagen deposition

4. Two patients are referred to the pulmonary diagnostic laboratory on the same day for pulmonary function testing. The first patient has advanced amyotrophic lateral sclerosis (ALS), while the second has idiopathic pulmonary fibrosis. If you were to compare the pulmonary function tests obtained in these two patients, which of the following measurements would you expect to fall within the normal range in the patient with ALS and abnormal range in the patient with pulmonary fibrosis?
A. Diffusion capacity for carbon monoxide
B. Forced expiratory volume in 1 second
C. Forced vital capacity
D. FEV_1/FVC
E. Total lung capacity

5. A 59-year-old woman with chronic obstructive pulmonary disease presents to the emergency department after developing the sudden onset of pleuritic left-sided chest pain and dyspnea. While she is being evaluated, she develops worsening dyspnea, tachycardia, and hypotension. On examination, her neck veins are distended, her trachea is deviated to the right, and she has absent breath sounds on the left side of her chest. Which of the following interventions is indicated at this time?

A. Electrocardiogram
B. Inhaled bronchodilators
C. Mechanical ventilatory support
D. Needle decompression of the left chest
E. Systemic corticosteroids

6. A 62-year-old woman is evaluated in the pulmonary clinic for a persistent dry cough and worsening dyspnea on exertion over an 18-month period. On examination, her oxygen saturation is 96% breathing air and falls to 90% when she walks around the clinic. She has crepitations on auscultation of the bilateral lower lung fields but no other significant findings. A chest radiograph shows low lung volumes and reticular opacities in the bilateral lower lobes, while a chest CT scan shows honeycombing and alveolar septal thickening in the bilateral lower lobes. Which of the following patterns would you expect to see on pulmonary function testing in this patient?

Choice	FEV$_1$	FVC	FEV$_1$/FVC%	TLC	DLCO
A	Normal	Normal	Normal	Normal	Normal
B	Normal	Normal	Normal	Normal	Decreased
C	Decreased	Decreased	Decreased	Increased	Decreased
D	Decreased	Decreased	Normal	Decreased	Decreased
E	Decreased	Decreased	Normal	Decreased	Increased

7. After being diagnosed with anterior uveitis by an ophthalmologist, a 38-year-old man is found to have bilateral hilar lymphadenopathy without parenchymal opacities on chest radiography and prolongation of the PR interval on an electrocardiogram. He is then referred to a pulmonologist who performs bronchoscopy with transbronchial biopsies, which demonstrate noncaseating granulomas. Which of the following is the most appropriate treatment for this patient?
A. Antifibrotic agent
B. Continued observation
C. Inhaled antimuscarinic
D. Inhaled long-acting β_2 agonist
E. Systemic corticosteroids

8. After presenting with worsening dyspnea on exertion over the past 18 months, a 63-year-old man who resides at sea level is referred for pulmonary function testing, which reveals the following:

Parameter	Predicted	Measured	% Predicted
FVC (liters)	4.00	2.16	54
FEV₁ (liters)	2.61	1.67	64
FEV₁/FVC	0.65	0.77	N/A
TLC (liters)	6.55	4.04	66
RV (liters)	2.54	1.88	74
DLCO (mL/min/mm Hg)	23.60	8.87	38

On evaluation in clinic, his oxygen saturation at rest is 94% while breathing air and he has bilateral crackles on lung examination. A chest radiograph reveals low lung volumes with net-like opacities in the lung bases, while a chest CT shows traction bronchiectasis (dilatation) and enlarged airspaces surrounded by thickened tissue in the periphery of the lung. Which of the following is the primary cause of the observed resting oxygen saturation?
A. Decreased cardiac output
B. Diffusion impairment
C. Hypoventilation
D. Shunt
E. Ventilation–perfusion mismatch

9. A 48-year-old woman presents with progressive shortness of breath on exertion and nonproductive over an 8-month period. She is a business executive, has never smoked, and owns two pet cockatiels. On examination, she has an S_pO_2 of 90% breathing air, scattered end-inspiratory crackles, and no clubbing. After pulmonary function testing reveals an FEV₁ 70% predicted, FVC 72% predicted, FEV₁/FVC 0.84, TLC 74% predicted, and DLCO 41% predicted, she undergoes a plain chest radiograph, which demonstrates bilateral interstitial (reticular) opacities more prominent in the upper lung zones. Which of the following would you expect to find on an arterial blood gas in this patient?
A. Acute respiratory alkalosis
B. Compensated respiratory acidosis
C. Compensated respiratory alkalosis
D. Metabolic acidosis with respiratory compensation
E. Metabolic alkalosis with respiratory compensation

10. A patient presents with chronic dyspnea on exertion and fatigue and undergoes pulmonary function testing. The results are shown in the table below.

Parameter	Predicted	Measured	% Predicted
FEV$_1$/FVC	0.81	0.84	N/A
TLC (liters)	5.9	3.9	67
DLCO (mL/min/mm Hg)	26.8	22.1	82
Maximum inspiratory pressure (cm H$_2$O)	−100	−40	40
Maximum expiratory pressure (cm H$_2$O)	120	110	91

Which of the following diagnoses is most consistent with the results observed on pulmonary function testing?
A. Diaphragmatic weakness
B. Duchenne muscular dystrophy
C. Hypersensitivity pneumonitis
D. Idiopathic pulmonary fibrosis
E. Sarcoidosis

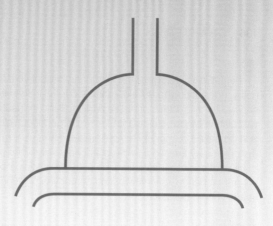

Pulmonary Vascular Diseases

6

The pathophysiology of the pulmonary vasculature is of great importance and takes many forms including development of edema in the interstitial and alveolar spaces due to changes in hydrostatic pressure and capillary permeability; obstruction of the pulmonary vasculature by blood clots that form in large, deep veins and travel to the lungs; and increased pulmonary arterial pressure and abnormal communications between the pulmonary arteries and the pulmonary veins. The pathophysiology and clinical manifestations vary between each of these entities, but they each have significant effects on gas exchange, mechanics, and hemodynamic function. At the end of this chapter, the reader should be able to:

- Describe the underlying mechanisms of the primary forms of cardiogenic and noncardiogenic pulmonary edema
- Describe the pathogenesis of pulmonary embolism
- Outline the effects of pulmonary edema and pulmonary embolism on lung mechanics, gas exchange, and the pulmonary circulation
- Describe the pathophysiological mechanisms of pulmonary hypertension
- Interpret clinical data to identify patients with idiopathic pulmonary arterial hypertension and arteriovenous malformations

PULMONARY EDEMA

Pulmonary edema is an abnormal accumulation of fluid in the interstitial and alveolar spaces of the lung. It is an important complication of a variety of heart and lung diseases and may be life-threatening.

Pathophysiology

Figure 5.1 reminds us that the pulmonary capillary is lined by endothelial cells and surrounded by an interstitial space. As the figure shows, the interstitium is narrow on one side of the capillary, where it is formed by the fusion of the two basement membranes, while on the other side, it is wider and contains type I collagen fibers. This latter region is particularly important for fluid exchange. Between the interstitial and alveolar spaces are the alveolar epithelium, composed predominantly of type 1 cells, and the superficial layer of surfactant (not shown in Figure 5.1).

The capillary endothelium is highly permeable to water and many solutes, including small molecules and ions. Proteins have a restricted movement across the endothelium. By contrast, the alveolar epithelium is much less permeable, and even small ions are largely prevented from crossing by passive diffusion. Water is actively pumped from the alveolar to the interstitial space by way of sodium channels and sodium–potassium ATPases located, respectively, in the alveolar apical and basolateral membranes.

Hydrostatic forces tend to move fluid out of the capillary into the interstitial space, and osmotic forces tend to keep it in. The movement of fluid across the endothelium is governed by the Starling equation:

$$\dot{Q} = K\left[(P_c - P_i) - \sigma(\pi_c - \pi_i)\right]$$ (Eq. 6.1)

where $\dot{Q}$ is the net flow out of the capillary; K is the filtration coefficient; P_c and P_i are the hydrostatic pressures in the capillary and interstitial space, respectively; π_c and π_i are the corresponding colloid osmotic pressures; and σ is the reflection coefficient. This last variable indicates the effectiveness of the membrane in preventing (reflecting) the passage of proteins compared with that of water across the endothelium and is reduced in diseases that damage the cells and increase permeability.

Although this equation is valuable conceptually, its practical use is limited. Of the four pressures, only one, the colloid osmotic pressure within the capillary, is known with any certainty. Its value is 25 to 28 mm Hg. The capillary hydrostatic pressure is probably halfway between arterial and venous pressures but varies markedly from top to bottom of the upright lung. The colloid osmotic pressure of the interstitial fluid is not known but is approximately 20 mm Hg in lung lymph. However, there are some questions as to whether this lymph has the same protein concentration as the interstitial fluid around the capillaries. The interstitial hydrostatic pressure is unknown but is thought by some physiologists to be substantially below atmospheric pressure. The value of σ in the pulmonary capillaries is approximately 0.7. It is probable that the net pressure from the Starling equilibrium is outward, causing a lymph flow of perhaps 20 mL/h.

The fluid that leaves the capillaries moves within the interstitial space of the alveolar wall and tracks to the perivascular and peribronchial interstitium (Figure 6.1). This tissue normally forms a thin sheath around the pulmonary arteries, veins, and bronchi and contains the lymphatics. The alveoli themselves are devoid of lymphatics, but once the fluid reaches the perivascular and peribronchial interstitium, some of it is carried in the lymphatics, while some moves through the loose interstitial tissue. The lymphatics actively pump the lymph toward the bronchial and hilar lymph nodes.

If excessive amounts of fluid leak from the capillaries, two factors tend to limit this flow. The first is a fall in the colloid osmotic pressure of the interstitial fluid as the protein is diluted as a result of the faster filtration of water compared with protein. However, this factor does not operate if the permeability of the capillary is greatly increased. The second is a rise in hydrostatic pressure in the interstitial space, which reduces the net filtration pressure.

Two stages in the formation of pulmonary edema are recognized (Figure 6.1). The first is *interstitial edema*, which is characterized by the engorgement of the perivascular and peribronchial interstitial tissue (cuffing), as shown in Figure 6.2. Widened lymphatics can be seen, and lymph flow increases. In addition, some widening of the interstitium of the thick side of the capillary occurs. Pulmonary function is little affected at this stage, and the condition is difficult to recognize, although some radiologic changes may be seen (see later text).

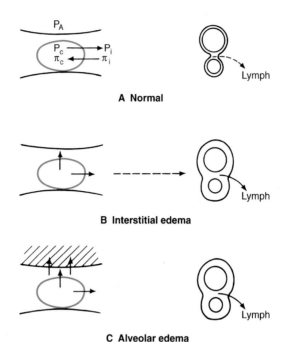

A Normal

B Interstitial edema

C Alveolar edema

Figure 6.1. Stages of pulmonary edema. A. There is normally a small lymph flow from the lung. **B.** Interstitial edema. Here there is an increased flow with engorgement of the perivascular and peribronchial spaces and some widening of the alveolar wall interstitium. **C.** Some fluid crosses the epithelium, producing alveolar edema.

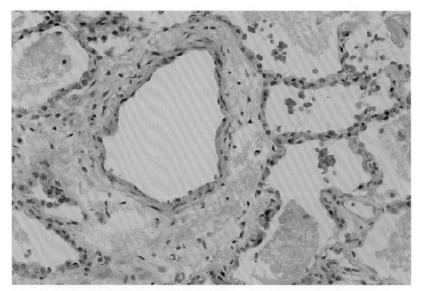

Figure 6.2. Example of engorgement of the perivascular space of a small pulmonary blood vessel by interstitial edema. Some alveolar edema is also present. (Image courtesy of Edward Klatt, MD.)

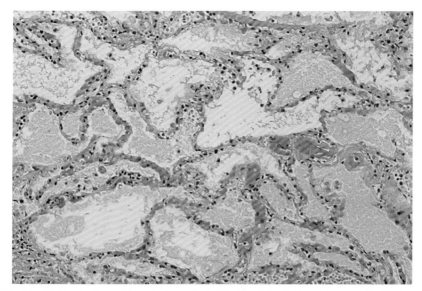

Figure 6.3. **Section of human lung showing alveolar edema.** (Image courtesy of Edward Klatt, MD.)

The second stage is *alveolar edema* (Figure 6.3). Here fluid moves across the epithelium into the alveoli, which are filled one by one. As a result of surface tension forces, the edematous alveoli shrink. Ventilation is prevented, and to the extent that the alveoli remain perfused, shunting of blood occurs and hypoxemia is inevitable. The edema fluid may move into the small and large airways and be coughed up as voluminous frothy sputum. The sputum is often pink because of the presence of red blood cells. Opacities are readily seen on chest radiographs (Figure 6.4). What prompts the transition from interstitial to alveolar edema is not fully understood, but it may be that the lymphatics

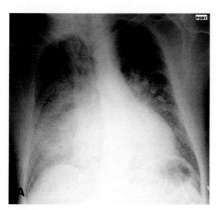
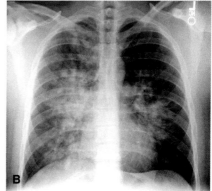

Figure 6.4. **Examples of pulmonary edema on plain chest radiography. A.** Pulmonary edema due to heart failure with reduced ejection fraction. **B.** High-altitude pulmonary edema. Note the difference in the size of the heart between the two images. (**B** image courtesy of Peter Hackett, MD.)

become overloaded and that the pressure in the interstitial space increases so much that fluid spills over into the alveoli. The alveolar epithelium may also be damaged and its permeability increased. This would explain the presence of protein and red cells in the alveolar fluid.

States of Pulmonary Edema

1. Interstitial edema

   Increased lymph flow from the lung

   Perivascular and peribronchial cuffing

   Septal lines on the chest radiograph

   Little effect on pulmonary function

2. Alveolar edema

   Often severe dyspnea and orthopnea

   Patients may cough up pink, frothy fluid

   Marked opacification on the radiograph

   Often severe hypoxemia

Pathogenesis

The underlying mechanisms for pulmonary edema and clinical situations in which they play a role are listed in Table 6.1. Any given clinical cause of pulmonary edema may develop as a result of one or several of these underlying mechanisms, with increases in capillary hydrostatic pressure or capillary permeability playing the most important roles. Reduced lymphatic drainage and

Table 6.1   Causes of Pulmonary Edema

Mechanism	Clinical Situations
Increased capillary hydrostatic pressure	Cardiogenic pulmonary edema (e.g., myocardial infarction, mitral stenosis, heart failure), neurogenic pulmonary edema, pulmonary venoocclusive disease
Increased capillary permeability	Toxin-mediated injury (inhaled or circulating), sepsis, radiation, oxygen toxicity, ARDS, transfusion-related acute lung injury
Reduced lymph drainage	Increased central venous pressure, lymphangitic carcinomatosis
Decreased interstitial pressure	Reexpansion pulmonary edema, negative pressure pulmonary edema
Decreased colloid osmotic pressure	Excessive administration of intravenous fluids, hypoalbuminemia

decreased colloid osmotic pressure rarely cause edema on their own but exaggerate the problems when another precipitating factor is present.

The protein and red blood cell concentrations of the edema fluid vary based on degree to which increased capillary permeability plays a role. When edema develops due to moderately increased hydrostatic pressure, the permeability characteristics of the capillary wall are preserved and the edema fluid has a low protein and red cell concentration. This is referred to as low permeability edema. When capillary permeability increases, however, due to either overly large rises in hydrostatic pressure or other factors, large amounts of protein and red blood cells are lost from the capillaries and the alveolar fluid has high protein and red blood cell concentrations.

Clinical Causes of Pulmonary Edema

The clinical causes of pulmonary edema can be grouped into one of two categories, cardiogenic and noncardiogenic.

Cardiogenic Pulmonary Edema

A variety of conditions affecting left heart function, including acute myocardial infarction, aortic and mitral valvular disease, and heart failure with reduced or preserved ejection fraction, cause increased left atrial pressure, which, in turn, raises pulmonary venous and capillary hydrostatic pressure and disturbs the Starling equilibrium. This can be recognized at right heart catheterization by measuring the pulmonary arterial wedge pressure (the pressure in a catheter that has been wedged in a small pulmonary artery), which is approximately equal to pulmonary venous pressure. If the pressure rises to sufficiently high levels, ultrastructural changes occur in the capillary walls, including disruption of the capillary endothelium and/or alveolar epithelium, resulting in increased permeability with movement of fluid, protein, and cells into the alveolar spaces. This phenomenon is known as capillary stress failure.

Whether pulmonary edema occurs with the cardiac problems noted above depends on the rate of rise of the hydrostatic pressure. For example, in patients in whom mitral valve dysfunction develops over a period of years, remarkably high pulmonary venous and capillary pressure may occur without clinical evidence of edema. This is partly because the caliber or number of the lymphatics increases to accommodate the higher lymph flow. However, these patients often have marked interstitial edema. By contrast, smaller but sudden increases in pulmonary venous and capillary pressure, as can occur following myocardial infarction or acute mitral valve dysfunction, typically lead to frank alveolar edema and rapid onset of respiratory failure.

Noncardiogenic Pulmonary Edema

There are a variety of situations in which pulmonary edema develops in the absence of left heart dysfunction.

High-Altitude Pulmonary Edema Affecting individuals traveling to altitudes above 2,400 m, high-altitude pulmonary edema develops as a result of excessive hypoxic pulmonary vasoconstriction and marked increases in pulmonary artery pressure. Current evidence shows that the arteriolar constriction is uneven and that regions of the capillary bed that are not protected from the high pressure develop increased permeability and, ultimately, the ultrastructural changes of stress failure (Figure 6.4B). Given the role of excessive hypoxic pulmonary vasoconstriction, pulmonary vasodilating medications such as calcium channel blockers and phosphodiesterase inhibitors can be used for prevention and treatment. Descent to lower elevation also plays a key role in treatment, as the increase in barometric pressure and alveolar P_{O_2} releases hypoxic pulmonary vasoconstriction and lowers pulmonary artery pressure.

Acute Respiratory Distress Syndrome Discussed in further detail in Chapter 8, acute respiratory distress syndrome (ARDS) is a severe form of lung injury that occurs in response to a variety of problems including pulmonary and nonpulmonary sepsis, aspiration, pancreatitis, trauma, smoke inhalation, and burns. An intense host cytokine–mediated inflammatory response contributes to edema formation by increasing capillary permeability and inhibiting active alveolar epithelial fluid reabsorption. Because this is a high permeability form of edema, the edema fluid typically has a high concentration of protein and red blood cells.

Reexpansion Pulmonary Edema Unilateral pulmonary edema can develop due to overly rapid reexpansion of a collapsed lung following pneumothorax or pleural effusion. The risk of this is highest when the duration of collapse exceeds 3 days. The mechanism is not clear but may relate to marked decreases in interstitial pressure when excessive negative pleural pressures are generated during drainage of the pneumothorax or effusion. High mechanical stresses in the alveolar walls may also contribute by causing ultrastructural changes in the capillary walls that increase capillary permeability.

Negative Pressure Pulmonary Edema Also referred to as postobstructive pulmonary edema, this form of edema develops after relief of severe upper airway obstruction. The mechanism is not entirely clear but may relate to decreases in interstitial pressure resulting from the extreme negative pleural pressures generated due to the intense effort to move air through the obstructed airway. The edema fluid typically has a low protein concentration, suggesting that the imbalance in hydrostatic forces is the primary factor rather than changes in permeability.

Neurogenic Pulmonary Edema Pulmonary edema can also develop following severe central nervous system injuries, including traumatic brain injury and subarachnoid hemorrhage. The mechanism is probably stress failure of pulmonary capillaries due to a large rise in capillary pressure resulting from a surge in sympathetic nervous system activity after the primary neurologic injury.

Opiate-Induced Pulmonary Edema Pulmonary edema can also complicate overdoses with both injected and orally administered opioids such as heroin and methadone. The high protein content of the edema fluid suggests this occurs due to increases in capillary permeability but the mechanism for these changes in permeability is not clear. Salicylate intoxication is another example of pulmonary edema complicating a substance overdose.

Pulmonary Venoocclusive Disease This is a rare form of pulmonary hypertension marked by fibrosis and subsequent narrowing or obliteration of the pulmonary veins in which edema develops as a result of increased pulmonary venous and capillary hydrostatic pressure. Fluid accumulation can be exacerbated by administration of pulmonary vasodilating medications that preferentially dilate the pulmonary arterioles and increase blood flow to the pulmonary capillaries. Further increases in hydrostatic pressure occur because of the difficulty maintaining flow against the high resistance of the pulmonary venous system.

Transfusion-Related Acute Lung Injury Occurring within 6 hours of red blood cell transfusion, this high permeability form of edema develops as a result of a complex array of factors including activation of the neutrophils sequestered in the lung microvasculature by antibodies or other components of the donated blood. A low permeability form of edema can also be seen if hydrostatic pressure rises too much following red blood cell transfusion in patients with impaired cardiac function.

Clinical Features

The clinical features of pulmonary edema vary to some extent based on the etiology of the edema, but some generalizations can be made. Dyspnea is the most common symptom. Mild edema may only be associated with dyspnea on exertion, whereas more severe edema is typically marked by dyspnea at rest. Orthopnea (increased dyspnea while recumbent) is common, particularly in patients with a cardiac etiology, as is paroxysmal nocturnal dyspnea (awakening at night with severe dyspnea and wheezing). Dry cough can be seen in the early stages, whereas in fulminant edema, patients may cough up large quantities of pink foamy sputum.

On examination, patients may have a rapid shallow breathing pattern. Fine end-inspiratory crepitations are heard at the lung bases in early edema. In more severe cases, musical sounds may also be heard because of airway narrowing, a phenomenon sometimes referred to as "cardiac asthma." Heart murmurs, increased jugular venous pulsation, and lower extremity edema may also be appreciated in patients with cardiogenic edema. Cyanosis may be present when edema leads to severe hypoxemia.

Findings on chest radiography vary depending on the underlying cause and extent of the edema. Interstitial edema causes septal lines to appear on the radiograph. Referred to as Kerley B lines, these are short, linear, horizontal markings originating near the pleural surface in the lower zones that are caused by edematous interlobular septa. Alveolar edema is marked by the presence of bilateral fluffy white opacities (Figure 6.4). Sometimes, these opacities radiate from the hilar regions, giving a so-called bat's-wing or butterfly appearance. The explanation of this distribution is not clear but may be related to the perivascular and peribronchial cuffing that is particularly noticeable around the large vessels in the hilar region (Figures 6.1 and 6.2). Cardiogenic edema is often accompanied by an enlarged heart, prominent pulmonary vessels, and pleural effusions (Figure 6.4A). These features are absent in noncardiogenic edema (Figure 6.4B).

Pulmonary Function

Extensive pulmonary function tests are seldom carried out on patients with pulmonary edema because they are so sick and the information is not necessary for diagnosis or treatment. The most important abnormalities are in the areas of mechanics and gas exchange.

Mechanics

Pulmonary edema reduces the distensibility of the lung and moves the pressure–volume curve downward and to the right (compare Figure 3.1). An important factor in this is the alveolar flooding, which causes a reduction in volume of the affected lung units as a result of surface tension forces and reduces their participation in the pressure–volume curve. In addition, interstitial edema per se probably stiffens the lung by interfering with its elastic properties, although it is difficult to obtain clear evidence on this. Edematous lungs require abnormally large expanding pressures during mechanical ventilation and tend to collapse to abnormally small volumes when not actively inflated (see Chapter 10).

Airway resistance is typically increased, especially if some of the larger airways contain edema fluid. Reflex bronchoconstriction due to stimulation of irritant receptors in the bronchial walls may also play a role. It is possible that in the absence of alveolar edema, interstitial edema increases the resistance of small airways as a result of their peribronchial cuff (Figure 6.1). This can be thought of as actually compressing the small airways or, at least, isolating them from the normal traction of the surrounding parenchyma (Figure 6.5). There is some evidence that this mechanism increases the closing volume (Figure 1.10) and thus predisposes to intermittent ventilation of the dependent lung.

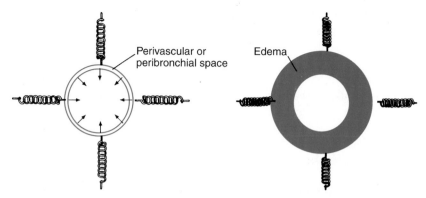

Figure 6.5. **Diagram showing how interstitial edema in the perivascular or peribronchial region can reduce the caliber of the vessel or airway.** The cuff isolates the structure from the traction of the surrounding parenchyma.

Gas Exchange

Interstitial edema has little effect on pulmonary gas exchange. A reduced diffusing capacity has sometimes been attributed to edematous thickening of the blood–gas barrier, but evidence for this is lacking. It is possible that cuffs of interstitial edema around small airways (Figures 6.1 and 6.5) can cause intermittent ventilation of dependent regions of the lung, leading to hypoxemia, but the importance of this in practice is uncertain.

Alveolar edema causes severe hypoxemia chiefly because of blood flow to unventilated units. These may be edema-filled alveoli or units supplied by airways that are completely obstructed by fluid. The shunt, which may be as much as 50% or more of the pulmonary blood flow in severe edema, can be reduced to some extent by hypoxic pulmonary vasoconstriction. Mechanical ventilation with PEEP often substantially reduces the amount of shunt by clearing edema fluid from some of the larger airways (see Figure 10.3), although it may not reduce total lung water.

Lung units with low ventilation–perfusion ratios also contribute to the hypoxemia. These presumably either lie behind airways that are partly obstructed by edema fluid or are units in which the ventilation is reduced by their proximity to edematous alveoli. Such lung units are particularly liable to collapse during treatment with oxygen-enriched mixtures (see Figures 9.4 and 9.5), but oxygen therapy is often essential to relieve the hypoxemia. Hypoxemia caused by edema can be exaggerated by decreased cardiac output and subsequent reductions in the mixed venous P_{O_2}, as can be seen with myocardial infarction or other cardiac problems.

The arterial P_{CO_2} is often normal or low in pulmonary edema because of increased ventilation to the nonedematous alveoli. This is provoked in part by the arterial hypoxemia and also possibly by stimulation of lung receptors (see next section). However, in fulminant pulmonary edema, carbon dioxide retention and respiratory acidosis may develop as a result of respiratory muscle fatigue.

Control of Ventilation
The rapid, shallow breathing often seen in pulmonary edema may be caused by stimulation of J receptors in the alveolar walls and perhaps other vagal afferents. The rapid breathing pattern minimizes the abnormally high elastic work of breathing. Arterial hypoxemia is an additional stimulus to breathing via the peripheral chemoreceptors.

Pulmonary Circulation
Pulmonary vascular resistance rises due to a combination of hypoxic pulmonary vasoconstriction in poorly or nonventilated areas and perivascular cuffing and increased resistance of the extra-alveolar vessels (Figures 6.2 and 6.5). Other possible factors are the partial collapse of edematous alveoli and alveolar wall edema that may compress or distort capillaries.

The topographical distribution of blood flow is sometimes altered by interstitial edema. The normal apex-to-base gradient becomes inverted, with the result that apical flow exceeds basal (Figure 6.6). This is most commonly seen in patients with mitral stenosis. The cause is not fully understood, but it is possible that perivascular cuffs particularly increase the resistance of the lower zone vessels because the lung is less well expanded there (see Figure 3.3). This inverted distribution is not seen in noncardiogenic forms of edema, such as ARDS.

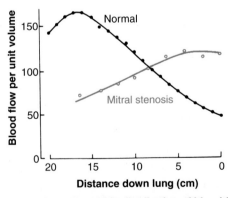

Figure 6.6. **Inversion of the topographic distribution of blood flow in a patient with mitral stenosis.** The cause is not certain, but interstitial cuffs of edema around the lower zone vessels (Figures 6.2 and 6.5) may be partly responsible.

PULMONARY EMBOLISM

Pulmonary embolism occurs when thrombi form in large veins and travel to the lungs where they become lodged in and occlude the pulmonary circulation. It is associated with significant morbidity and mortality and can be challenging to diagnose.

Pathogenesis

The majority of responsible thrombi arise from the deep veins of the lower extremities, but they may also originate in the upper extremities, right side of the heart, and the pelvic veins. Nonthrombotic emboli, such as fat, air, and amniotic fluid, also occur in very specific circumstances but are less common than venous thrombi.

Venous thrombi tend to form in the setting of three important conditions, often referred to as Virchow's triad:

1. Stasis of blood
2. Alterations in the blood coagulation system (hypercoagulability)
3. Abnormalities of the vessel wall (intimal injury)

Stasis of blood is promoted by immobilization following a fracture, severe illness, acute spinal cord injury, surgery, local pressure, or venous obstruction.

The intravascular *coagulability of blood* is increased in several conditions, such as polycythemia vera and sickle cell disease, which increase the viscosity of the blood leading to sluggish flow next to the vessel wall. A variety of genetic conditions affecting the coagulation cascade are now recognized including antithrombin 3 deficiency, factor V Leiden mutation, hyperhomocysteinemia, and proteins C and S deficiency. Other conditions, including widespread malignancy, pregnancy, nephrotic syndrome, and use of oral contraceptives are also associated with hypercoagulability, but the mechanism for these changes is not entirely clear. Aside from genetic and other testing to identify some of the hypercoagulable states listed above, there is no reliable method to identify an increased tendency for intravascular coagulation.

The *vessel wall may be damaged* by local trauma or by inflammation. This is a common mechanism for venous thrombi following pelvic and lower extremity fractures or surgery, for example. Where there is marked local phlebitis with tenderness, redness, warmth, and swelling, the clot may be more securely adherent to the wall.

When the thrombus fragment is released, it is rapidly swept into one of the pulmonary arteries. While very large thrombi become lodged in a large artery, the thrombus may break up and block several smaller vessels. The lower lobes are frequently involved because they have a high blood flow (see Figure 3.3).

Pulmonary infarction, that is, death of the embolized tissue, occurs infrequently. More often there is distal hemorrhage and atelectasis, but the alveolar structures remain viable. Depletion of alveolar surfactant may contribute to these changes. Infarction is more likely if the embolus completely blocks a large artery or if there is preexisting lung or heart disease. Infarction results in alveolar filling with extravasated red cells and inflammatory cells and causes opacity on the radiograph. Rarely, the infarct becomes infected, leading to an abscess. The infrequency of infarction can be explained, in part, by the fact that most emboli do not obstruct the vessel completely. In addition, bronchial artery anastomoses and the airways supply oxygen to the lung parenchyma.

Clinical Features

The presentation depends considerably on the size of the embolus and the patient's preexisting cardiopulmonary status.

Small Emboli

While small emboli may present with dyspnea and chest pain, they are frequently unrecognized or only detected as an incidental finding on chest imaging studies performed to evaluate other problems. Repeated small emboli can gradually obliterate the pulmonary capillary bed, resulting in pulmonary hypertension (described further below).

Medium-Sized Emboli

These often present with acute onset of dyspnea and pleuritic pain and, less commonly, slight fever and cough productive of blood-streaked sputum. Tachycardia is common, and on auscultation there may be a pleural friction rub. A small pleural effusion may develop. Embolism may mimic pneumonia, although the two entities can typically be distinguished by the rapidity of symptom onset, which is faster for pulmonary embolism.

Massive Emboli

These present with signs of hemodynamic collapse including pallor, shock, loss of consciousness, or cardiac arrest. The pulse is rapid and weak, the blood pressure is low, and the neck veins are engorged.

Thrombosis in the deep veins of the legs or pelvis is often unsuspected until embolism occurs. Asymmetric swelling of the lower extremities is an important finding but is not always present. Local tenderness, calf pain on dorsiflexion of the ankle, or other signs of inflammation may or may not be present.

Features of Pulmonary Embolism for Different-Sized Emboli

Small emboli

Frequently unrecognized

Repeated emboli may result in pulmonary hypertension

Medium-sized emboli

Sometimes pleuritic pain, dyspnea, and slight fever

Cough may produce blood-stained sputum

May produce pleural friction rub

Chest radiograph is often normal or nearly so

Massive emboli

Hemodynamic collapse with shock, pallor, and cardiac arrest

Hypotension with rapid, weak pulse and neck vein engorgement

Sometimes fatal

Diagnosis

Due to the wide variability in clinical presentation, pulmonary embolism can be very difficult to diagnose. The most common finding on electrocardiography is a nonspecific sinus tachycardia, but evidence of right heart strain may also be present. Chest radiography is typically unrevealing, although in rare cases, peripheral wedge-shaped opacities suggestive of infarction or areas of decreased vascular markings (oligemia) may be seen. Contrast-enhanced CT scans of the chest are the most commonly used diagnostic test, with the key finding being the presence of filling defects in the pulmonary vasculature (Figure 6.7). For patients who cannot undergo CT scanning due to the

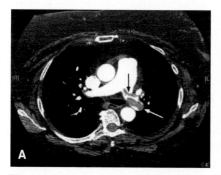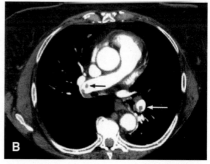

Figure 6.7. Examples of pulmonary emboli on contrast-enhanced CT scan of the chest. Emboli are detected by showing areas where contrast does not fill the pulmonary vasculature, referred to as a "filling defect." **A.** The *black arrow* points to a filling defect in the proximal left main pulmonary artery, while the *white arrow* points to a filling defect further out in the left main pulmonary artery. **B.** The *black arrow* points to a filling defect in the right main pulmonary artery, while the *white arrow* demonstrates a filling defect in the left lower lobe pulmonary artery.

risk of contrast administration, lung scans can be made after injecting radio-labeled albumin aggregates into the venous circulation and comparing the distribution of perfusion with the distribution of ventilation measured following inhalation of a radio-labeled aerosol (Figure 6.8). Pulmonary angiography is considered the diagnostic gold standard but is not widely used due to the invasiveness of the procedure and the increasing quality of CT scans. When the diagnosis is suspected based on clinical features, but chest imaging is not available or feasible, a presumptive diagnosis of pulmonary embolism can be made by identifying deep venous thrombosis with duplex ultrasonography of the upper and lower extremities. This is not effective for examining the iliac or pelvic veins, however.

Pulmonary Function

Pulmonary Circulation

This normally has a large reserve capacity because many capillaries are unfilled. When the pulmonary artery pressure rises on exercise, for example, these capillaries are recruited and, in addition, some capillary distention occurs. This reserve means that at least half of the pulmonary circulation can be obstructed by an embolus before there is a substantial rise in pulmonary artery pressure.

In addition to the purely mechanical effects of the embolus, there is some evidence that active vasoconstriction occurs, at least for some minutes after embolization (Figure 6.9). The mechanism is not understood, but in experimental animals, local release of serotonin from platelets associated with the embolus has been implicated, as well as reflex vasoconstriction via the sympathetic nervous system. It is not known to what extent these factors operate in humans.

If the embolus is large and if the pulmonary artery pressure rises considerably, the right ventricle may begin to fail. The end-diastolic pressure increases, arrhythmias may develop, and the tricuspid valve may become incompetent. Rarely, pulmonary edema can be seen, presumably due to leakage from those capillaries not protected from the raised pulmonary artery pressure (Compare with high-altitude pulmonary edema).

The increase in pulmonary artery pressure gradually subsides over the subsequent days as the embolus resolves. This occurs both through fibrinolysis and through organization of the clot into a small fibrous scar attached to the vessel wall. Patency of the vessel is thus usually restored. As noted above, repeated small emboli over time can lead to chronic thromboembolic pulmonary hypertension.

Mechanics

When a pulmonary artery is occluded by a catheter in humans and experimental animals, the ventilation to that area of lung is reduced. The mechanism appears to be a direct effect of the reduced alveolar P_{CO_2} on the smooth muscle

VENTILATION
R   L

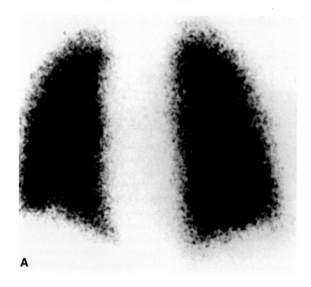

A

PERFUSION
R   L

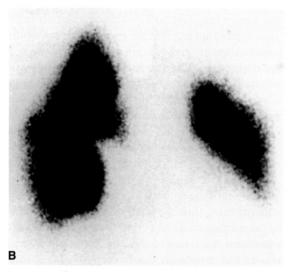

B

Figure 6.8. **Ventilation–perfusion scan in a patient with multiple pulmonary emboli. A.** The ventilation image (made with xenon-133) shows a normal pattern. **B.** The perfusion image (made with technetium-99m albumin) shows areas of absent blood flow in both lungs.

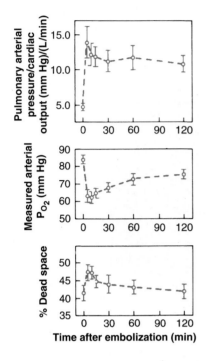

Figure 6.9. Transient changes in pulmonary artery pressure (related to cardiac output), arterial P_{CO_2}, and physiologic dead space in dogs following experimental thromboembolism. These suggest active responses of the pulmonary circulation and airways. The importance of these mechanisms in humans is unknown. (Reprinted with permission from Dantzker DR, Wagner PD, Tornabene VW, et al. Gas exchange after pulmonary thromboembolization in dogs. *Circ Res*. 1978L;42:92–103.)

of the local small airways, causing bronchoconstriction. It can be reversed by adding carbon dioxide to the inspired gas.

Although this airway response to vascular obstruction is generally much weaker than the corresponding vascular response to airway obstruction (hypoxic vasoconstriction), it serves a similar homeostatic role. The reduction in airflow to the unperfused lung reduces the amount of wasted ventilation and thus the physiologic dead space. This mechanism is apparently short-lived or ineffective after pulmonary thromboembolism in humans because most measurements of the distribution of ventilation with radioactive xenon made some hours after the episode show no defect in the embolized area. However, in experimental animals, transient changes in alveolar P_{O_2}, physiologic dead space, and airway resistance often occur after thromboembolism (Figure 6.9).

The elastic properties of the embolized region may change some hours after the event. In experimental animals, ligation of one pulmonary artery is followed by patchy hemorrhagic edema and atelectasis in the affected lung within 24 hours. This has been attributed to the loss of pulmonary surfactant, which has a rapid turnover and apparently cannot be replenished in a lung that has lost its pulmonary blood flow. Again, it is not yet clear how often this occurs in human pulmonary thromboembolism or whether it is part of the pathological process that has been traditionally called infarction. The fact that most emboli do not completely block the vessel presumably limits its occurrence.

Gas Exchange

Moderate hypoxemia without carbon dioxide retention is often seen after pulmonary embolism. Measurements by the multiple inert gas elimination technique show that the hypoxemia is primarily explained by ventilation–perfusion inequality. Both the physiologic shunt and dead space are increased, as demonstrated in Figure 6.10, which shows distributions from two patients after

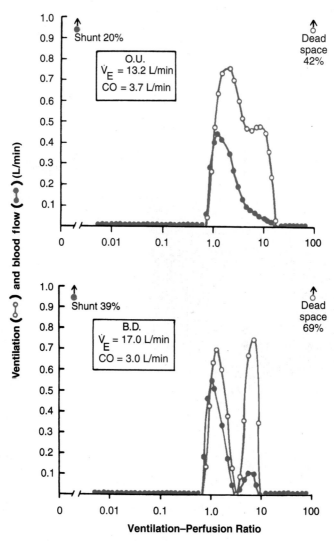

Figure 6.10. Distributions of ventilation–perfusion ratios in two patients with acute massive pulmonary embolism. Note that in both instances, the hypoxemia could be explained by large shunts (blood flow to unventilated lung). In addition, there was a large increase in ventilation to lung units with abnormally high ventilation–perfusion ratios representing the embolized regions. (Reprinted from D'Alonzo GE, Bower JS, DeHart P, et al. The mechanisms of abnormal gas exchange in acute massive pulmonary embolism. *Am Rev Respir Dis*. 1983;128(1):170–172. Copyright © 1983 American Thoracic Society. All Rights Reserved.)

massive pulmonary embolism. The most striking features are the large shunts (blood flow to unventilated alveoli) of 20% and 39% and the existence of lung units with high ventilation–perfusion ratios. The latter feature can be explained by the embolized regions where the blood flow is typically greatly reduced but not abolished completely. The precise mechanism of the shunts is not certain, but it may be blood flow through the areas of hemorrhagic atelectasis.

Another important cause of ventilation–perfusion mismatch is redistribution of blood flow to the nonembolized areas of the lung. Because the entire cardiac output must traverse the pulmonary circulation, blood that would normally go through occluded regions must now travel through other lung units thus reducing their ventilation–perfusion ratio and depressing the arterial P_{O_2}. Other explanations for the hypoxemia have been advanced, including diffusion impairment in areas with ongoing blood flow and therefore reduced transit time (see Figure 2.4) and opening up of latent pulmonary artery–vein anastomoses as a consequence of the high pulmonary artery pressure.

Following pulmonary embolism, the arterial P_{CO_2} is maintained at the normal level by increasing the ventilation to the alveoli (see Figure 2.10). The increase in ventilation may be substantial because of the large physiologic dead space, and therefore wasted ventilation, caused by the embolized areas. Decreased arterial P_{CO_2} is occasionally seen when patients raise ventilation more than necessary to compensate for the increased physiologic dead space in response to pain and anxiety. Increased arterial P_{CO_2} is uncommon but can occur in patients who lack the ability to raise ventilation, as can happen with severe underlying lung disease or in select patients receiving invasive mechanical ventilation.

Differences can be seen in P_{CO_2} between arterial blood and end-tidal gas. The mixed alveolar P_{CO_2} tends to be low because of the high $\dot{V}_A/\dot{Q}$ in the embolized region. Because there is little uneven ventilation in this disease, the end-tidal P_{CO_2} approximates the mixed alveolar value and is also reduced. Identification of this arterial end-tidal P_{CO_2} difference has been suggested as a diagnostic tool for pulmonary embolism but is not part of standard diagnostic algorithms.

PULMONARY HYPERTENSION

The normal mean pulmonary artery pressure is approximately 15 mm Hg; an increased level (greater than 25 mm Hg) is called pulmonary hypertension.

Pathogenesis

Three principal mechanisms are as follows:

1. *Increased Pulmonary Vascular Resistance.* Normal pulmonary vascular resistance is less than 3 mm Hg/min/L. Increased values can be seen due to several mechanisms:

a. Structural changes in the blood vessels including medial hypertrophy, intimal thickening, and plexiform lesions. These changes occur in the pulmonary arterioles and lead to narrowing of the vessels and increased resistance. This is the primary mechanism in patients with idiopathic pulmonary arterial hypertension (see below) as well as pulmonary hypertension seen in patients with scleroderma, systemic lupus erythematosus, cirrhosis, human immunodeficiency virus, and methamphetamine abuse.

b. Vasoconstriction, principally because of alveolar hypoxia, as occurs in long-term residents at high altitude or the obesity hypoventilation syndrome. This is also a contributor to pulmonary hypertension in severe obstructive lung disease.

c. Vascular obstruction, as in chronic thromboembolism. In addition, the vessels may be occluded by circulating fat, air, amniotic fluid, or cancer cells. In schistosomiasis, the parasites lodge in small arteries and cause a granulomatous reaction, which narrows the vessel lumen. A similar phenomenon can occur when talc particles contaminate illicit substances injected by people who abuse drugs.

d. Obliteration of the pulmonary capillary bed, as in emphysema (see Figures 4.2 and 4.3) or idiopathic pulmonary fibrosis. Various forms of arteritis can also occur, such as in polyarteritis nodosa. Rarely, the small veins are involved, as in pulmonary venoocclusive disease.

2. *Increased Left Atrial Pressure.* Seen in patients with mitral valve disease or left ventricular failure, this is a very common cause of pulmonary hypertension. Although the changes in pulmonary artery pressure are due to a high left atrial and pulmonary venous pressure, sustained increases in pressure can cause structural changes in the walls of the small pulmonary arteries, including medial hypertrophy and intimal thickening, which increase pulmonary vascular resistance.

3. *Increased Pulmonary Blood Flow.* This occurs in congenital heart diseases with left-to-right shunts through ventricular or atrial septal defects or a patent ductus arteriosus. Initially, the rise in pulmonary artery pressure is relatively small because of the ability of the pulmonary capillaries to accommodate high flows by recruitment and distension. However, sustained high flows result in structural changes in the walls of the small arteries. If left untreated, pulmonary artery pressure may reach systemic levels, reversing the direction of the shunt and causing arterial hypoxemia (Eisenmenger's syndrome).

Clinical Presentation and Diagnosis

The clinical presentation varies significantly depending on the underlying etiology. If the clinical picture suggests pulmonary hypertension, echocardiography is typically performed to estimate the pulmonary artery systolic pressure by determining the amount of regurgitation through the tricuspid valve. Right heart catheterization is the gold standard for measuring pulmonary artery pressure but is invasive and often not required. Once pulmonary hypertension is confirmed on these tests, additional testing is done to determine the etiology, which serves as a guide for treatment.

Idiopathic Pulmonary Arterial Hypertension

This is an uncommon disorder of uncertain cause, although in some cases a genetic predisposition is present. Pulmonary artery pressure is increased due to increased pulmonary vascular resistance resulting from medial hypertrophy, intimal thickening, and plexiform arteriopathy (Figure 6.11). It typically occurs in young to middle-aged women and usually presents with dyspnea on exertion, although in more severe cases, syncope or chest pain on exertion may occur. Physical examination may demonstrate a right ventricular heave, a loud pulmonic component of the second heart sound, a murmur of tricuspid regurgitation, increased jugular venous distention, and lower extremity edema. Electrocardiography demonstrates right axis deviation and other signs of right ventricular hypertrophy while plain chest radiography may show enlarged pulmonary arteries and signs of right atrial and ventricular enlargement. Patients often have hypoxemia, particularly on exertion, and a decreased diffusing capacity for carbon monoxide. When suspected based on

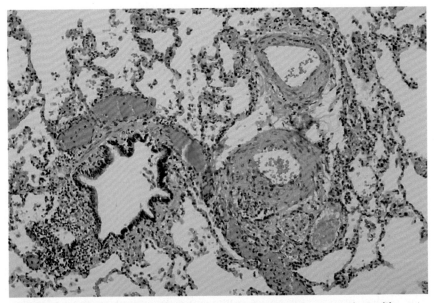

Figure 6.11. Section of human lung obtained on autopsy from a patient with idiopathic pulmonary arterial hypertension. Note the increased thickness of the wall of the arterioles due to smooth muscle hypertrophy. The vessel lumen is narrowed leading to increased vascular resistance. (Image courtesy of Edward Klatt, MD.)

the findings noted above and echocardiography, the diagnosis is confirmed by identifying increased pulmonary vascular resistance and normal left atrial pressure on right heart catheterization. Left untreated, the disease progresses inexorably and is associated with very high mortality within just a few years. Recent advances in pharmacologic therapy, however, including the use of oral and intravenous pulmonary vasodilators, have led to significant improvements in patient outcomes.

Cor Pulmonale

This term refers to right heart disease secondary to primary disease of the lung. The occurrence of right ventricular hypertrophy and fluid retention in COPD was discussed in Chapter 4. The same findings may occur late in severe restrictive lung disease.

The various factors that lead to pulmonary hypertension include obliteration of the capillary bed by the destruction of alveolar walls or interstitial fibrosis; obstruction by thromboemboli, hypoxic pulmonary vasoconstriction, and hypertrophy of smooth muscle in the walls of the small arteries; and increased viscosity of the blood caused by polycythemia. Whether the term "right heart failure" should be applied to all these patients is disputed. In some, the output of the heart is increased because it is operating high on the Starling curve, and the output can increase further on exercise. The principal physiological abnormality in these patients is fluid retention. However, in others, true right heart failure develops. Some physicians restrict the term cor pulmonale to those patients who have electrocardiographic evidence of right ventricular hypertrophy.

PULMONARY ARTERIOVENOUS MALFORMATION

This uncommon condition is characterized by an abnormal communication between a branch of a pulmonary artery and vein. Most patients have hereditary hemorrhagic telangiectasias. As implied by the name of the disease, these patients also have telangiectasias of the skin or mucous membranes, suggesting the presence of a general vascular defect, and often have a personal or family history of recurrent epistaxis or gastrointestinal bleeding due to vascular abnormalities on those mucosal surfaces as well. In addition to telangiectasias, some patients have finger clubbing and a bruit may be detected on auscultation over the fistula.

Small lesions cause no functional disturbances, whereas larger fistulae cause true shunts and hypoxemia. The arterial P_{O_2} is depressed far below the expected value during oxygen breathing (see Figure 2.6). Because the arteriovenous malformations are often located in the lower portions of the lung, flow through the malformations and shunt increases when patients are in the upright position.

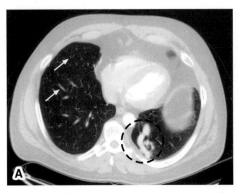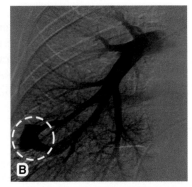

Figure 6.12. Pulmonary arteriovenous malformation (AVM) on chest CT **(A)** and pulmonary angiography **(B)**. **A.** The *black dotted circle* outlines the AVM in the left lower lobe. The size of this vessel can be compared to normal vessels highlighted by the *white arrows* in the right lung. **B.** The *white dotted circle* outlines the AVM. Note the difference in size compared to other vessels in the periphery of the lung.

This accounts for the fact that patients with large fistulae report dyspnea that is worse when upright (platypnea) and experience a decline in oxygen saturation when they move from the supine to upright position (orthodeoxia). While large arteriovenous malformations can be seen on plain chest radiography, contrast-enhanced CT scans are the preferred diagnostic test (Figure 6.12). Large, untreated arteriovenous malformations increase the risk of cerebrovascular accidents and intracerebral abscess due to the loss of the filter function of the pulmonary capillary network. This risk is minimized by embolizing large arteriovenous malformations using interventional radiology.

KEY CONCEPTS

1. Fluid movement across the pulmonary capillary endothelium is determined by the Starling equation, and disturbances of the normal equilibrium can result in pulmonary edema. A common cause is an increase in capillary pressure as a result of left heart failure.

2. Clinical features of pulmonary edema include dyspnea, orthopnea, cough with blood-stained sputum, tachycardia, and crepitations on auscultation.

3. Two stages of pulmonary edema are recognized: interstitial and alveolar. The first is difficult to detect, but the second causes major symptoms and signs.

4. Pulmonary embolism is frequently undiagnosed. Medium-sized emboli typically cause pleuritic pain, dyspnea, and cough with blood-streaked sputum, while massive emboli cause cardiopulmonary collapse. A CT angiogram of the chest is diagnostic.

5. Pulmonary hypertension can be caused by an elevated venous pressure as in left heart failure, an increase in pulmonary blood flow as in some congenital heart diseases, or an increase in pulmonary vascular resistance as in idiopathic pulmonary arterial hypertension, long-term residents at high altitude, chronic thromboembolism, and loss of capillaries in emphysema or pulmonary fibrosis.

CLINICAL VIGNETTE

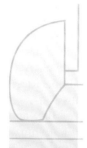

A 72-year-old woman underwent surgical repair of a pelvic fracture suffered during a fall at home. After the surgery, she did well while undergoing physical therapy in anticipation of discharge to a rehabilitation facility. On the fourth hospital day, she developed acute onset of left-sided pleuritic chest pain and dyspnea while trying to get up to move from her bed to a chair. Upon examination, she had a blood pressure of 113/79 mm Hg, heart rate of 117 beats per minute, a respiratory rate of 22 breaths per minute, and oxygen saturation of 90% breathing air. She was using accessory muscles of respiration but had clear breath sounds on auscultation. Her cardiac exam was normal except for her regular tachycardia and she had bilateral leg edema that was greater on the right than on the left. An arterial blood sample drawn while breathing air showed a P_{CO_2} of 39 mm Hg and P_{O_2} of 61 mm Hg. An electrocardiogram showed sinus tachycardia but no ischemic changes. A portable chest radiograph showed no focal opacities, effusions, or pneumothorax. A CT pulmonary angiogram was obtained and showed filling defects in the left lower lobe pulmonary artery.

Questions

- What risk factor(s) predisposed the patient to this problem?
- If you were to perform echocardiography, what changes would you expect to see in her pulmonary artery pressure and right heart function?
- How do you account for the fact that she has a normal P_{CO_2} on her arterial blood sample?
- What is the mechanism for the patient's hypoxemia?

QUESTIONS

For each question, choose the best answer.

1. A 41-year-old man presents with a sudden onset of severe dyspnea accompanied by pleuritic left-sided chest pain that began several hours after a transoceanic flight. There is no fever, cough, or hemoptysis.

On examination, he has clear breath sounds on auscultation, and a normal cardiac examination but leg edema that is greater on the right than on the left. Which is the most appropriate initial diagnostic test?
A. Bronchoscopy
B. CT of the chest with contrast
C. Echocardiogram
D. Pulmonary angiography
E. Spirometry

2. A 61-year-old woman with no history of smoking is admitted to the hospital with 2 days of worsening dyspnea and a nonproductive cough. On examination, her blood pressure was normal, she had an elevated jugular venous pulsation, a third heart sound, no murmurs, diffuse crepitations on lung auscultation, and bilateral leg edema. A chest radiograph showed cardiomegaly and diffuse bilateral opacities, while an echocardiogram performed shortly following admission showed a dilated left ventricle with a low ejection fraction of 30% and an increased estimated pulmonary artery systolic pressure of 50 mm Hg. Which of the following most likely accounts for her pulmonary hypertension?
A. Granulomatous inflammation in the pulmonary arterioles
B. Increased left atrial and pulmonary venous pressure
C. Increased pulmonary blood flow
D. Medial hypertrophy and intimal thickening of the pulmonary arterioles
E. Occlusion of the pulmonary vascular bed by recurrent thromboemboli

3. A previously healthy 22-year-old woman who has spent 3 days in a high-altitude mountain hut at 4,500 m develops severe dyspnea with minimal exertion and a cough productive of pink-tinged sputum. Her oxygen saturation by pulse oximetry is found to be abnormally low. Auscultation reveals bilateral crackles in both lungs. Which of the following mechanisms is most likely responsible for this woman's condition?
A. Decreased colloid osmotic pressure
B. Decreased interstitial pressure
C. Endotoxin-mediated increase in capillary permeability
D. Exaggerated hypoxic pulmonary vasoconstriction
E. Increased left atrial pressure

4. A 57-year-old man with known very severe COPD who continues to smoke cigarettes presents to his doctor with increasing weight gain and bilateral lower leg edema over several weeks. On examination, he has an elevated jugular venous pulsation and bilateral lower leg edema that extends to his knees. An electrocardiogram shows right ventricular

hypertrophy and right axis deviation. Which of the following is the most appropriate diagnostic test at this time?
A. Bronchoscopy
B. CT scan of the chest without contrast
C. Duplex ultrasonography of the lower extremities
D. Echocardiography
E. Spirometry

5. A 41-year-old man presents for evaluation of worsening dyspnea over several months. He notes that his dyspnea is worse in the upright position and reports intermittent epistaxis but denies cough, fever, or hemoptysis. His family history is notable for a father and brother with recurrent gastrointestinal bleeding. On exam, his oxygen saturation is 95% while supine and 89% when upright. He has scattered telangiectasias on his ears and in his nasolabial folds but no crackles or wheezes. The results of arterial blood gases performed while breathing air and an F_IO_2 of 1.0 in the seated position are shown below:

F_IO_2	Arterial P_{O_2} (mm Hg)
0.21	60
1.0	300

For which of the following complications is this individual at risk without appropriate treatment?
A. Cerebrovascular accident
B. Cor pulmonale
C. Pulmonary edema
D. Pulmonary fibrosis
E. Pulmonary hypertension

6. A 64-year-old man with a history of hypertension and coronary artery disease presents to the emergency department with several hours of markedly worsening dyspnea. On exam, he is afebrile and has an oxygen saturation of 90% breathing air. He is laboring to breathe, has an increased jugular venous pulsation, a laterally displaced point of maximal impulse, diffuse bilateral crackles on lung exam, and bilateral pitting lower extremity edema, which the patient states is worse than normal. A chest radiograph demonstrates a large heart shadow with bilateral alveolar opacities in a perihilar distribution. Which of the following changes in pulmonary function would you expect to find at the time of his presentation to the emergency department?

A. Decreased closing volume
B. Decreased elastic recoil of the lung
C. Increased airway resistance
D. Increased diffusing capacity for carbon monoxide
E. Increased lung compliance

7. Four days after undergoing a total left hip arthroplasty, a 74-year-old man develops acute onset of dyspnea and right-sided chest pain. His vitals include a temperature of 36.5°C, heart rate of 95 beats per minute, respiratory rate of 24 breaths per minute, and oxygen saturation of 89% breathing air. He has clear breath sounds on auscultation, a rapid, but regular heart rate, no murmur and 2+ right lower extremity edema. An arterial blood gas while breathing air demonstrates pH of 7.38, P_{CO_2} of 39 mm Hg, and P_{O_2} of 60 mm Hg. A CT scan of the chest with intravenous contrast is obtained and a representative image is shown in the figure below.

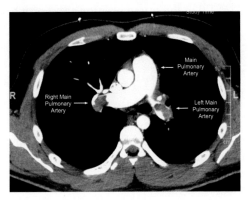

Which of the following mechanisms best explains the observed oxygen saturation in this patient?
A. Decreased alveolar ventilation relative to CO_2 production
B. Increased airway secretions
C. Left-to-right shunt through a patent foramen ovale
D. Redistribution of blood flow leading to areas of low ventilation–perfusion ratios
E. Thickening of the alveolar capillary barrier

8. A 45-year-old woman is evaluated for worsening dyspnea on exertion over a 6-month period. She has no other significant medical problems aside from a 20-pack year smoking history. On examination, she has elevated neck veins, clear breath sounds, a loud second heart sound, no murmur, and trace bilateral lower extremity edema. Pulmonary function testing reveals an FEV_1/FVC of 0.82 and a diffusing capacity for carbon

monoxide of 53% predicted. Chest radiography demonstrates large pulmonary arteries and right ventricular enlargement, but no opacities or effusions. On right heart catheterization, she has a mean pulmonary artery pressure of 33 mm Hg, pulmonary vascular resistance of 5.2 mm Hg/min/L (normal: less than 3 mm Hg/min/L), and a pulmonary artery occlusion pressure of 8 mm Hg (normal 2 to 12 mm Hg). Which of the following is the most likely cause of this patient's presentation?

A. Arteriovenous malformation
B. Chronic obstructive pulmonary disease
C. Mitral stenosis
D. Pulmonary arterial hypertension
E. Ventricular septal defect

9. Four days following an anterior wall myocardial infarction, a previously healthy 51-year-old man develops acute onset of dyspnea and hypoxemia. On exam, he has a new, loud holosystolic murmur that was not present on admission. A chest radiograph is obtained and is shown below. An echocardiogram is performed and reveals severe mitral regurgitation.

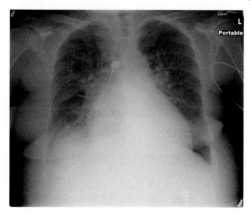

Which of the following mechanisms most likely accounts for the observed hypoxemia and findings on chest radiography?

A. Decreased interstitial colloid osmotic pressure
B. Increased interstitial hydrostatic pressure
C. Increased lymphatic drainage
D. Increased pulmonary capillary colloid osmotic pressure
E. Increased pulmonary capillary hydrostatic pressure

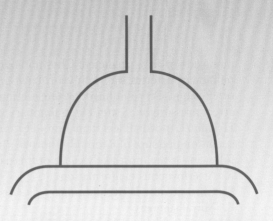

Environmental, Occupational, Neoplastic, and Infectious Diseases

7

In the previous three chapters, we considered three categories of lung diseases—obstructive diseases, restrictive diseases, and pulmonary vascular diseases—that each has characteristic pathophysiology. There are a range of other problems that can affect the lungs and cause derangements in pulmonary function but do not necessarily fall neatly into one of these categories. They are the focus of this chapter. At the end of this chapter, the reader should be able to:

- Describe the main atmospheric pollutants and their effects on the respiratory system
- Predict the location and method of airway deposition based on the size of an aerosol
- Describe the primary mechanisms for clearing deposited particles
- Use clinical, radiographic, and pulmonary function data to identify the major pneumoconioses
- Describe the potential effects of pulmonary neoplasms on pulmonary function
- Describe the clinical features and effects on pulmonary function of pulmonary infections and cystic fibrosis

DISEASES CAUSED BY INHALED PARTICLES

Many occupational and industrial lung diseases are caused by inhaled dusts. Atmospheric pollutants are also important factors in the etiology of other diseases, such as chronic bronchitis, emphysema, asthma, and bronchial carcinoma, so we will start by looking at the environment in which we all live.

Atmospheric Pollutants

Carbon Monoxide

This is the largest pollutant by weight in the United States (Figure 7.1, *left*). It is produced by the incomplete combustion of carbon in fuels, chiefly in the automobile engine (Figure 7.1, *right*). The main hazard of carbon monoxide is its propensity to bind to hemoglobin. Because carbon monoxide has more than 200 times the affinity of oxygen, it competes successfully with this gas for hemoglobin binding sites. Carbon monoxide also increases the oxygen affinity of the remaining hemoglobin with the result that it does not release its oxygen so readily to the tissues and can inhibit mitochondrial cytochrome oxidase (See *West's Respiratory Physiology: The Essentials*, 11th ed., p. 99-100). Commuters using a busy urban freeway may have 5% to 10% of their hemoglobin bound to carbon monoxide, particularly if they smoke cigarettes. The emission of carbon monoxide and other pollutants by automobile engines can be reduced by installing a catalytic converter that processes the exhaust gases.

Nitrogen Oxides

These are produced when fossil fuels (coal, oil) are burned at high temperatures in power stations and automobiles. These gases cause inflammation of

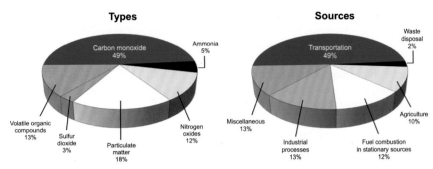

Figure 7.1. **Air pollutants (by weight) in the United States.** Volatile organic compounds refers to hydrocarbons that are volatile and can convert to the gaseous phase at room temperature and atmospheric pressure. Particulate matter refers to particles 10 micrometers and smaller. Figures derived using data from the 2017 National Emissions Inventory, United States Environmental Protection Agency.

the eyes and upper respiratory tract during smoggy conditions. At higher concentrations, they can cause acute tracheitis, acute bronchitis, and pulmonary edema. The yellow haze of smog is a result of these gases.

Sulfur Oxides

These are corrosive, poisonous gases produced when sulfur-containing fuels are burned, chiefly by power stations. These gases cause inflammation of the mucous membranes, eyes, upper respiratory tract, and bronchial mucosa. Short-term exposure to high concentrations causes pulmonary edema. Long-term exposure to lower levels results in chronic bronchitis in experimental animals. The best way to reduce emissions of sulfur oxides is to use low-sulfur fuels.

Hydrocarbons

Hydrocarbons, like carbon monoxide, represent unburned wasted fuel. They are not toxic at concentrations normally found in the atmosphere. However, they are hazardous because they form photochemical oxidants under the influence of sunlight (discussed below).

Particulate Matter

This includes particles with a wide range of sizes, up to visible smoke and soot. Major sources are power stations and industrial plants. Often emission of polluting particles can be reduced by processing the waste air stream by filtering or scrubbing, although removing the smallest particles is often expensive.

Photochemical Oxidants

These include ozone and other substances, such as peroxyacyl nitrates, aldehydes, and acrolein. They are not primary emissions but are produced by the action of sunlight on hydrocarbons and nitrogen oxides. These reactions are slow with the result that the concentration of the photochemical oxidants may increase several kilometers from where the oil was released. Photochemical oxidants cause inflammation of the eyes and respiratory tract, damage to vegetation, and offensive odors. In higher concentrations, ozone causes pulmonary edema. These oxidants contribute to the thick haze of smog.

The concentration of atmospheric pollutants is often greatly increased by a temperature inversion, that is, a low layer of cold air beneath warmer air. This prevents the normal escape of warm surface air with its pollutants to the upper atmosphere. The deleterious effects of a temperature inversion are particularly marked in low-lying areas surrounded by hills, such as the Los Angeles basin. Exposure to atmospheric pollutants is typically higher in large urban centers. As a result, the burden of disease from such exposures falls heavily on residents of these areas, often underrepresented minorities, which likely contributes significantly to observed disparities in the prevalence and outcomes of some forms of lung disease.

Major Atmospheric Pollutants

- Carbon monoxide
- Nitrogen oxides
- Sulfur oxides
- Hydrocarbons
- Particulate matter
- Photochemical oxidants

Cigarette Smoke

This is one of the most important pollutants in practice because it is inhaled by smokers in concentrations many times greater than the pollutants in the atmosphere. It includes approximately 4% carbon monoxide, enough to raise the carboxyhemoglobin level in a smoker's blood to 10%, a percentage sufficient to impair exercise and cognitive performance. The smoke also contains the highly addictive alkaloid nicotine, which stimulates the autonomic nervous system, causing tachycardia, hypertension, and sweating. Aromatic hydrocarbons and other substances, loosely called "tars," are apparently responsible for the high risk of bronchial carcinoma in cigarette smokers. A male who smokes 35 cigarettes per day has 40 times the risk of a nonsmoker. Increased risks of chronic bronchitis, emphysema, coronary artery disease, and peripheral arterial disease are also well documented.

Electronic cigarettes have been proposed as an alternative method for delivering nicotine without the risks of combustible tobacco. Given the relatively short duration of their commercial availability, the long-term effects on pulmonary function and risk of lung cancer remain unclear, although some evidence suggests that electronic cigarettes cause similar disruptions in the protease–antiprotease balance as combustible tobacco, which could predispose to development of emphysema. Widespread use among teenagers has become a significant public health issue, including concerns about the risk of early nicotine addiction and potential for conversion to combustible tobacco.

Deposition of Aerosols in the Lung

The term *aerosol* refers to a collection of small particles that remains airborne for a substantial amount of time. Many pollutants exist in this form, and their pattern of deposition in the lung depends chiefly on their size. The properties of aerosols are also important in understanding the fate of inhaled bronchodilators. Three mechanisms of deposition are recognized.

Impaction
Impaction refers to the tendency of the largest inspired particles to fail to turn the corners of the respiratory tract. As a result, many particles impinge on the mucous surfaces of the nose and pharynx (Figure 7.2A) and also on the bifurcations of the large airways. Once a particle strikes a wet surface, it is trapped and not subsequently released. The nose is remarkably efficient at removing the largest particles by this mechanism; almost all particles greater than 20 μm in diameter, and approximately 95% of particles 5 μm in diameter are filtered by the nose during resting breathing. Figure 7.3 shows that most of the deposition of particles over 3 μm in diameter occurs in the nasopharynx during nose breathing.

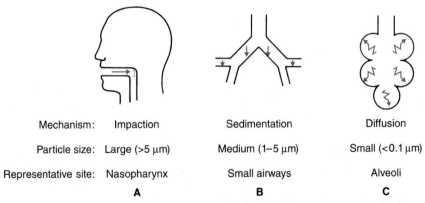

Mechanism:	Impaction	Sedimentation	Diffusion
Particle size:	Large (>5 μm)	Medium (1–5 μm)	Small (<0.1 μm)
Representative site:	Nasopharynx	Small airways	Alveoli
	A	**B**	**C**

Figure 7.2. Scheme of deposition of aerosols in the lung. The term *representative sites* does not mean that these are the only sites where this form of deposition occurs. For example, impaction also occurs in the medium-sized bronchi, and diffusion also occurs in the large and small airways. (See text for details.)

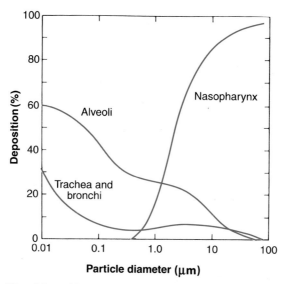

Figure 7.3. Site of deposition of aerosols. The largest particles remain in the nasopharynx, but some of the small particles can penetrate to the alveoli.

Sedimentation

Sedimentation is the gradual settling of particles because of their weight (Figure 7.2B). It is particularly important for medium-sized particles (1 to 5 μm). Deposition by sedimentation occurs extensively in the small airways, including the terminal and respiratory bronchioles. The chief reason is simply that the dimensions of those airways are small and therefore the particles have a shorter distance to fall. Note that the particles, unlike gases, are not able to diffuse from the respiratory bronchioles to the alveoli because of their negligibly small diffusion rate. (See *West's Respiratory Physiology: The Essentials*, 11th ed., p. 6).

An example of this phenomenon is the accumulations of dust around the terminal and respiratory bronchioles in early coal worker's pneumoconiosis (Figure 7.4). Although the retention of dust depends on both deposition and clearance, and it is possible that some of this dust was transported from peripheral alveoli, the appearance is a graphic reminder of the vulnerability of this region of the lung. It has been suggested that some of the earliest changes in chronic bronchitis and emphysema are secondary to the deposition of atmospheric pollutants (including tobacco smoke particles) in these small airways.

Diffusion

Diffusion is the random movement of particles as a result of their continuous bombardment by gas molecules (Figure 7.2C). It occurs to a significant extent only in the smallest particles (less than 0.1 μm in diameter). Deposition

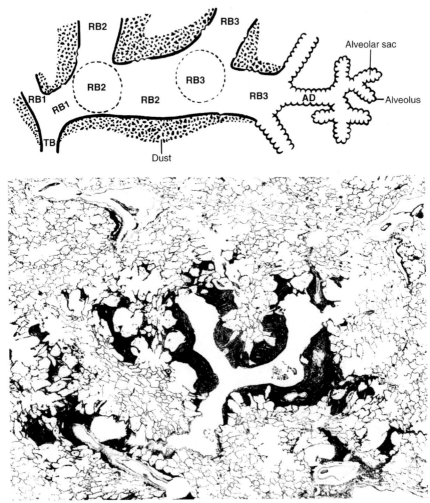

Figure 7.4. **Section of lung from a coal miner showing accumulations of dust around the respiratory bronchioles.** These small airways show some dilatation, sometimes called focal emphysema. (Reprinted from Heppleston AG, Leopold JG. Chronic pulmonary emphysema: Anatomy and pathogenesis. *Am J Med*. 1961;31:279–291. Copyright © 1961 Elsevier. With permission.)

by diffusion chiefly takes place in the small airways and alveoli where the distances to the wall are least. However, some deposition by this mechanism also occurs in the larger airways.

Many inhaled particles are not deposited at all but are exhaled with the next breath. In fact, only some 30% of 0.5-μm particles may be left in the lung during normal resting breathing. These particles are too small to impact or sediment to a large extent. In addition, they are too large to diffuse significantly. As a result, they do not move from the terminal and respiratory bronchioles to the alveoli by diffusion, which is the normal mode of gas movement in this region. Small particles may become larger during inspiration by aggregation or by absorbing water.

The pattern of ventilation affects the amount of aerosol deposition. Slow, deep breaths increase the penetration into the lung and thus increase the amount of dust deposited by sedimentation and diffusion. Exercise results in higher rates of airflow and, in particular, increases deposition by impaction. In general, deposition of dust is proportional to the ventilation during exercise, which is therefore an important factor during work in mines, for example.

Deposition and Clearance of Inhaled Particles

Deposition	Clearance
Impaction	Mucociliary system
Sedimentation	Alveolar macrophages
Diffusion	

Clearance of Deposited Particles

Fortunately, the lung is efficient at removing particles that are deposited within it. Two distinct clearance mechanisms exist: the mucociliary system and the alveolar macrophages (Figure 7.5).

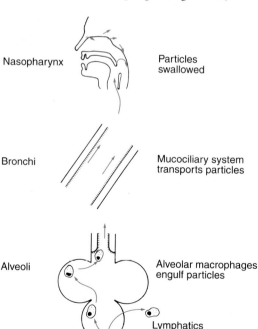

Nasopharynx — Particles swallowed

Bronchi — Mucociliary system transports particles

Alveoli — Alveolar macrophages engulf particles — Lymphatics

Figure 7.5. Clearance of inhaled particles from the lung. Particles that deposit on the surface of the airways are transported by the mucociliary escalator and swallowed. Particles that reach the alveoli are engulfed by macrophages, which either migrate to the ciliary surface or escape via the lymphatics.

Mucociliary System

Mucus is produced by two sources:

1. Bronchial seromucous glands situated deep in the bronchial walls (see Figures 4.6, 4.7, and 7.6). Both mucus-producing and serous-producing cells are present, and ducts lead the mucus to the airway surface.
2. Goblet cells, which form part of the bronchial epithelium.

The 5- to 10-μm thick layer of mucus assists in clearance of deposited material by two means. First, it contains the immunoglobulin IgA, which is derived from plasma cells and lymphoid tissue and is an important defense against foreign proteins, bacteria, and viruses. Second and perhaps more important is movement of the two-layer mucus toward the upper airway (Figure 7.6). Cilia beat within the deeper sol layer, which helps move the superficial gel layer in a cephalad direction. The gel layer is relatively tenacious and viscous, which aids in trapping deposited particles while the deeper sol layer is less viscous and thus allows cilia to beat within it easily.

The cilia are 5 to 7 μm long and beat in a synchronized fashion at between 1,000 and 1,500 times per minute. During the forward stroke, the tips of the cilia apparently come in contact with the gel layer, thus propelling it. However, during the recovery phase, the cilia are bent so much that they move entirely within the sol layer, where the resistance is less.

The mucous blanket moves up at around 1 mm/min in small peripheral airways but as fast as 2 cm/min in the trachea, and eventually the particles reach the level of the pharynx where they are swallowed or expectorated. The clearance of a healthy bronchial mucosa is essentially complete in less than 24 hours. In very dusty environments, mucous secretion may be increased so much that cough and expectoration assist in the clearance.

Abnormal retention of secretions occurs in some diseases due to abnormalities in ciliary function or due to changes in the composition of the mucus such that it cannot be propelled easily by the cilia. The former is seen in the ciliary dyskinesias while the latter occurs in cystic fibrosis and asthma.

The normal operation of the mucociliary system is also affected by pollution and disease. The cilia apparently can be paralyzed by the inhalation of toxic gases, such as oxides of sulfur and nitrogen, and perhaps by tobacco smoke. In acute inflammation of the respiratory tract, as, for example, following influenza infection, the bronchial epithelium may be denuded. Changes in the character of the mucus may occur with infection, thus making it difficult for the cilia to transport it. Mucous plugging of bronchi occurs in asthma, but the mechanism is unknown. Finally, in chronic infections such as bronchiectasis and chronic bronchitis, the volume of secretions may be so great that the ciliary transport system is overwhelmed.

Alveolar Macrophages

The mucociliary system stops short of the alveoli, and particles deposited there are engulfed by macrophages. These amoeboid cells roam around the surface of the alveoli. When they phagocytose foreign particles, they either migrate to the small airways where they load on to the mucociliary escalator (Figure 7.5) or they leave the lung in the lymphatics or possibly the blood. When the dust burden is large or the dust particles are toxic, some of the macrophages migrate through the walls of the respiratory bronchioles and dump their dust there. Figure 7.4 shows the accumulations of dust around the respiratory bronchioles in the lung of a coal miner. In the case of toxic dusts, such as silica, a fibrous reaction is stimulated in this region.

The macrophages not only transport bacteria out of the lung but also kill them in situ by means of the lysozymes they contain. As a consequence, the alveoli quickly become sterile, although it takes some time for the dead organisms to be cleared from the lung. Immunologic mechanisms are also important in the antibacterial action of macrophages. Normal macrophage activity can be impaired by various factors, such as cigarette smoke, oxidant gases such as ozone, alveolar hypoxia, radiation, administration of corticosteroids, and the ingestion of alcohol. Macrophages that engulf particles of silica are often destroyed by this toxic material.

Coal Worker's Pneumoconiosis

The term *pneumoconiosis* refers to parenchymal lung disease caused by inorganic dust inhalation. One form seen in coal workers is directly related to the amount of coal dust to which the miner has been exposed.

Pathology
Early and late forms of the disease should be distinguished. In simple coal worker's pneumoconiosis, coal dust macules (Figure 7.7A) can be seen, as can aggregations of coal particles around terminal and respiratory bronchioles,

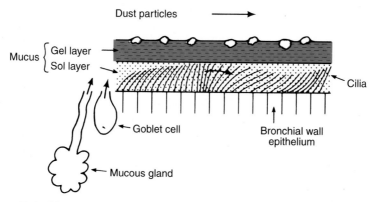

Figure 7.6. Mucociliary escalator. The mucous film consists of a superficial gel layer that traps inhaled particles and a deeper sol layer. It is propelled by cilia.

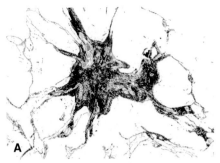 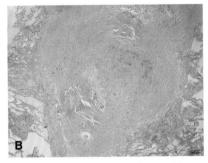

Figure 7.7. A. Coal dust macule with surrounding emphysema in an individual with simple coal worker's pneumoconiosis. (Image courtesy of Victor Roggli, MD.) **B.** A silicotic nodule in an individual with silicosis. (Image courtesy of the National Coal Workers' Autopsy study, Sidney Clingerman, BS and Ann F. Hubbs, DVM, PhD.)

with some dilatation of these small airways (Figure 7.4) In the advanced form, known as progressive massive fibrosis, condensed masses of black fibrous tissue infiltrated with dust are seen. Only a small fraction of miners exposed to heavy dust concentrations develop progressive massive fibrosis.

Clinical Features

Simple coal worker's pneumoconiosis apparently causes little disability despite its radiographic appearance. The dyspnea and cough that often accompany the disease are closely related to the smoking history of the miner and are probably chiefly caused by associated chronic bronchitis and emphysema. By contrast, progressive massive fibrosis usually causes increasing dyspnea and may terminate in respiratory failure.

The chest radiograph of simple pneumoconiosis shows a delicate micronodular mottling, and various stages in the advance of the disease are recognized depending on the density of the shadows. Progressive massive fibrosis results in large, irregular dense opacities often surrounded by abnormally radiolucent lung.

Pulmonary Function

Simple pneumoconiosis usually causes little functional impairment by itself. However, sometimes a small reduction in forced expiratory volume, an increase in residual volume (RV), and a fall in arterial P_{O_2} are seen. It is often difficult to know whether these changes are caused by associated chronic bronchitis and emphysema due to smoking.

Progressive massive fibrosis causes a mixed obstructive and restrictive pattern. Distortion of the airways results in irreversible obstructive changes, whereas the large masses of fibrous tissue reduce the useful volume of the lung. Increasing hypoxemia, cor pulmonale, and terminal respiratory failure may occur.

Silicosis

This pneumoconiosis is caused by the inhalation of silica (SiO_2) during quarrying, mining, or sandblasting. Whereas coal dust is virtually inert, silica particles are toxic and provoke a severe fibrous reaction in the lung.

Pathology
Silicotic nodules composed of concentric whorls of dense collagen fibers are found around respiratory bronchioles, inside alveoli, and along the lymphatics (Figure 7.7B). Silica particles may be seen in the nodules using polarized microscopy.

Clinical Features
Mild forms of the disease may cause no symptoms, while advanced disease results in cough and severe dyspnea, especially on exercise. Chest radiography in early disease shows fine nodular marking whereas more severe forms demonstrate streaks of fibrous tissue, and progressive massive fibrosis (Figure 7.8). The disease may progress long after exposure to the dust has ceased. In addition to an increased risk of lung cancer, patients with silicosis are at increased risk for tuberculosis and nontuberculous mycobacterial and fungal infections.

Pulmonary Function
The changes are similar to those seen in coal worker's pneumoconiosis but are often more severe. In advanced disease, generalized interstitial fibrosis may develop, with a restrictive type of defect, hypoxemia, particularly with exercise, and a reduced diffusing capacity.

Asbestos-Related Diseases

Asbestos is a naturally occurring fibrous mineral silicate that is used in a variety of industrial applications, including heat insulation, pipe lagging, roofing

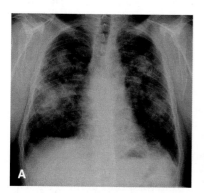
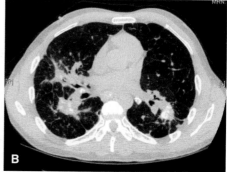

Figure 7.8. Chest imaging in progressive massive fibrosis. A. Plain chest radiograph demonstrating bilateral, patchy, confluent opacities. **B.** Single slice from a CT scan of the chest showing dense bilateral patchy opacities. The prominent white areas within the opacities represent calcification.

materials, and brake linings. Asbestos fibers are long and thin, and it is possible that their aerodynamic characteristics allow them to penetrate far into the lung. When they are in the lung, they may become encased in proteinaceous material. If these are coughed up in the sputum, they are known as asbestos bodies.

Three health hazards are recognized:

1. Pulmonary fibrosis (asbestosis): This develops gradually after heavy exposure and presents with progressive dyspnea (especially on exercise), weakness, finger clubbing, and fine basal crepitations. Chest radiography demonstrates basilar reticular opacities, which resemble those seen in idiopathic pulmonary fibrosis. The two can be distinguished by the fact that patients with asbestosis often have calcified asbestos plaques. Pulmonary function tests in advanced disease reveal a typical restrictive pattern with reductions of vital capacity and lung compliance. A fall in diffusing capacity occurs relatively early in the disease.
2. Bronchial carcinoma: The risk is greatly increased by concurrent cigarette smoking.
3. Pleural disease: This can present as pleural thickening and plaques, which are usually harmless, pleural effusions or malignant mesothelioma. Mesothelioma is an aggressive cancer that can develop as much as 40 years after exposure. It is associated with progressive restriction of chest movement, severe chest pain, and a rapid downhill course that is not very amenable to treatment.

Other Pneumoconioses

A variety of other dusts cause simple pneumoconiosis. Examples include iron and its oxides, which cause siderosis and result in a striking, mottled radiographic appearance. Antimony and tin are other culprits. Beryllium exposure results in granulomatous lesions of acute or chronic types with pulmonary manifestations, including interstitial fibrosis, that resemble those of sarcoidosis. The disease is now much less common than it was as a result of strict control of beryllium in industry.

Byssinosis

Some inhaled organic dusts cause airway reactions rather than alveolar reactions. A good example is byssinosis, which follows exposure to cotton dust, especially in the cardroom where the fibers are disentangled, cleaned, and then intermixed.

The pathogenesis is not fully understood, but it appears that the inhalation of some active component in the bracts (leaves around the stem of the cotton boll) leads to the release of histamine from mast cells in the lung. The resulting bronchoconstriction causes dyspnea and wheezing. A feature of the disease is that the symptoms are worse on entering the mill, especially after a period of absence. For this reason, it has been referred to as "Monday fever."

The symptoms resemble those of asthma and include dyspnea, tightness of the chest, wheezing, and an irritating cough. Workers who have already had chronic bronchitis or asthma are especially susceptible.

Pulmonary function tests show an obstructive pattern with reductions in FEV_1, FVC, FEV_1/FVC, and $FEF_{25\%-75\%}$. Airway resistance and inequality of ventilation are increased. Typically, these abnormalities gradually become worse over the course of the working day, but partial or complete recovery occurs during the night or over the weekend. There is no evidence of parenchymal involvement, and the chest radiograph is normal. However, epidemiologic studies show that daily exposure over 20 years or so causes permanent impairment of lung function of the type associated with chronic obstructive pulmonary disease (COPD).

Occupational Asthma

Various occupations involve exposure to allergenic organic dusts, and some individuals develop hypersensitivity. These individuals include flour mill workers who are sensitive to the wheat weevil, lumber industry workers exposed to western red cedar, printers exposed to gum acacia, and workers handling fur or feathers. Toluene diisocyanate (TDI) is a special case because some individuals develop an extreme sensitivity to this substance, which is used in the manufacture of polyurethane products. Similar to byssinosis, symptoms, signs, and abnormalities in pulmonary function may abate during time away from work.

NEOPLASTIC DISEASES

Bronchial Carcinoma

This book is about the function of the diseased lung and how this is reflected in pulmonary function tests. For neoplastic diseases, this is generally not an important topic because, with the exception of very advanced disease, the effects of lung cancer on pulmonary function are often minor compared to the more important issues of diagnosis, staging, and treatment. Accordingly, this section is relatively brief, and textbooks of pathology or internal medicine should be consulted for additional details on diagnosis, staging, and management of this disease.

Despite being a largely preventable disease, lung cancer continues to have a very high incidence and remains the leading cause of cancer mortality in both men and women in the United States.

Pathogenesis

There is overwhelming evidence that cigarette smoking is a major factor. Epidemiologic studies show that an individual who smokes 20 cigarettes a day has about 20 times the chance of dying from the disease than a nonsmoker of the same age and sex. Furthermore, risk decreases dramatically if the individual stops smoking.

The specific causative agents in cigarette smoke are uncertain, but many potential carcinogenic substances are present, including aromatic hydrocarbons, phenols, and radioisotopes. Many smoke particles are submicronic and penetrate far into the lung. However, the fact that many bronchogenic carcinomas originate in the large bronchi suggests that deposition by impaction or sedimentation may play an important role (Figure 7.2). Also, the large bronchi are exposed to a high concentration of tobacco smoke products as the material is transported from the more peripheral regions by the mucociliary system. Individuals who inhale other people's smoke (passive smokers) also have an increased risk. It is too early to know how electronic cigarettes affect the risk of lung cancer.

Other etiological factors are recognized. Urban dwellers are more at risk, suggesting that atmospheric pollution plays a part. This finding is hardly surprising in view of the variety of chronic respiratory tract irritants that exist in the air in urban environments (Figure 7.1). Occupational factors also exist, especially exposure to chromates, nickel, arsenic, asbestos, and radioactive gases.

Classification

Most pulmonary neoplasms fall within one of two categories: small cell and non–small cell carcinoma.

A. *Small cell carcinomas.* These contain a homogeneous population of oat-like cells giving a characteristic appearance. They are highly malignant and have often metastasized by the time of diagnosis. These tumors often present as large, central masses. They are seldom seen in peripheral lung and usually do not cavitate.

B. *Non–small cell carcinomas.* This is now the most common form of lung cancer and includes several subtypes.

1. *Adenocarcinomas* are the most common non–small cell carcinoma, with an increasing incidence, particularly among women. They typically occur in the periphery of the lung, show glandular differentiation, and often produce mucus.

2. *Squamous carcinomas* have a characteristic microscopic appearance, including intercellular bridges, keratin, and a whorl- or nest-like pattern to the cells. Most squamous cell cancers arise in the proximal airways, but peripheral lesions can be seen. Cavitation occurs sometimes with either central or peripheral lesions.

3. *Large cell carcinomas* are epithelial cancers that lack glandular or squamous features and thus cannot be classified as adenocarcinomas or squamous cell carcinomas. They tend to occur in the periphery of the lung and often demonstrate necrosis.

Bronchioalveolar carcinoma was a term formally used to describe a fourth type of non–small cell carcinoma marked by peripheral location, well-differentiated cytology, growth along alveolar septa, and the ability to spread via the airways or lymphatics. More recent classification schemes now place these tumors in one of several subcategories of adenocarcinoma such as adenocarcinoma in situ or minimally invasive adenocarcinoma.

Some tumors show a heterogeneity of cell type that makes classification difficult. There are also a variety of other pulmonary neoplasms, including carcinoid tumors and mesothelioma, that do not fall within this classification system.

Clinical Features and Diagnosis

Nonproductive cough and hemoptysis are common early symptoms, whereas weight loss is a sign of advanced disease. Tumors that compress the left recurrent laryngeal nerve can present with hoarseness, while dyspnea is seen with neoplasms that cause a large pleural effusion or bronchial obstruction. Depending on the size, location, and extent of the tumor, patients can have negative physical exams or lymphadenopathy and signs of lobar collapse, consolidation, or pleural effusion. The chest radiograph is useful for diagnosis, but small carcinomas may only be visible on CT scan of the chest or bronchoscopy. CT-guided biopsy, mediastinoscopy, and a variety of bronchoscopic techniques, including endobronchial ultrasound, are used to facilitate early diagnosis. Sputum cytology may be useful in a limited number of patients.

Pulmonary Function

While lung function is typically normal in early disease, it is often impaired in moderately advanced–severe disease. A large pleural effusion causes a restrictive defect, as may the collapse of a lobe after complete bronchial obstruction. Partial obstruction of a large bronchus can result in an obstructive pattern. The obstruction can be caused either by a tumor within the lumen of the airway or by compression by a mass or lymphadenopathy external to the airway. Sometimes the movement of the lung on the affected side is seen to lag behind that of the normal lung, and air may cycle back and forth between the normal and obstructed lobes (see *West's Respiratory Physiology: The Essentials*, 11th ed., p. 204). This cycle is known as pendelluft (swinging air). Complete obstruction of a mainstem bronchus typically yields a restrictive pattern with low FEV_1 and FVC but a normal FEV_1/FVC ratio.

Even though pulmonary function abnormalities are not a prominent feature of many pulmonary neoplasms, assessment of pulmonary function still plays a key role in the management of some patients. When tumors are amenable to surgical resection, patients undergo pulmonary function testing to determine whether they can tolerate the planned surgical procedure or require a less extensive resection.

INFECTIOUS DISEASES

Infectious diseases are of great importance in pulmonary medicine. However, aside from hypoxemia, they generally do not cause specific patterns of impaired pulmonary function, and pulmonary function tests are of little value in the evaluation of these patients. Since this book is about the function of the diseased lung and its measurement using pulmonary function tests, infectious diseases are not considered in great detail. A textbook on internal medicine or pathology should be consulted for further details.

Pneumonia

This term refers to inflammation of the lung parenchyma associated with alveolar filling by exudate. While this is most commonly due to infections with bacteria such as *Streptococcus pneumoniae* or *Legionella pneumophila*, it can also be seen with infections with viruses, including influenza and SARS-CoV-2, or fungi (discussed below).

Pathology
The alveoli are crammed with cells, chiefly polymorphonuclear leukocytes. Resolution often occurs with restoration of the normal morphology. However, suppuration may result in necrosis of tissue, causing a lung abscess. Special forms of pneumonia include that following aspiration of oral secretions or animal or mineral oil (lipoid pneumonia).

Clinical Features
These features vary considerably depending on the causative organism, the age of the patient, and his or her general condition. The usual features of bacterial pneumonia include malaise, fever, and cough that is often productive of purulent sputum. Pleuritic pain occurs when the pneumonia extends to the edge of the lung abutting the pleural surface. Examination reveals rapid shallow breathing, tachycardia, and sometimes cyanosis. Often there are signs of consolidation, and the chest radiograph shows opacification (Figure 7.9). This may involve all of a lobe (lobar pneumonia), but frequently the distribution is patchy and centered around the airways (bronchopneumonia). Viral pneumonias tend to cause diffuse bilateral opacities rather than focal consolidation. Parapneumonic effusions can develop in response to the pneumonia and, in some cases, become infected, a situation referred to as empyema. Sputum examination and culture frequently identify the causative organism, although some common causes of pneumonia, such as *Legionella* and mycoplasma, do not readily grow on routine culture media. In some cases, urine antigen studies are used to identify certain *Streptococcus* and *Legionella* species.

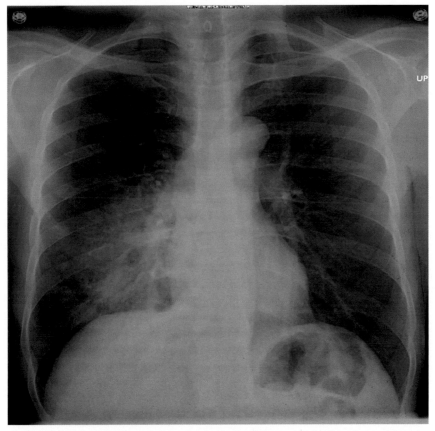

Figure 7.9. Chest radiograph from a patient with pneumonia. There is an opacity in the right lower lung zone.

Pulmonary Function

Because the pneumonic region is not ventilated, it causes shunt and hypoxemia. The severity of hypoxemia varies based on the amount of lung affected by the pneumonia and the local pulmonary blood flow, which may be substantially reduced either by the disease process itself or by hypoxic vasoconstriction. When pneumonia is complicated by the acute respiratory distress syndrome, severe hypoxemia and reduced compliance can be seen. Carbon dioxide retention does not generally occur in pneumonia due to increased ventilation to the uninvolved areas of lung, while chest movement may be restricted by pleural pain or by a pleural effusion.

Tuberculosis

Pulmonary tuberculosis (TB) takes many forms. Advanced disease is much less common now in many parts of the world because of improvements in public health and increasing availability of effective antituberculous drugs, although the disease remains common in places like sub-Saharan Africa, particularly among people infected with human immunodeficiency virus (HIV). Cases are still seen in high-income countries, however, due to the increasing ease of travel and frequency of immigration from TB-endemic regions.

Upon initial infection, referred to as primary TB, the majority of people remain asymptomatic, although some develop fever, parenchymal opacities, and hilar lymphadenopathy. Isolated pleural effusions may also be seen. Whether or not patients manifest symptoms, once the primary infection is controlled, bacilli often remain in the patient, contained within granulomas. This situation, referred to as latent TB infection, can be identified by a hypersensitivity response on TB skin testing or through assays that detect interferon gamma release from blood lymphocytes stimulated by TB antigens.

If cell-mediated immunity is preserved, most patients never develop active disease again. Individuals who have defects in cell-mediated immunity through, for example, HIV infection or use of immunosuppressive medications, can develop reactivation TB, which often presents with subacute onset of dyspnea, productive cough, hemoptysis, and constitutional symptoms along with upper lobe opacities, fibrosis and cavitation. Extensive fibrosis can lead to restrictive impairments in pulmonary function.

While effective treatments for tuberculosis are readily available, the emergence of multidrug-resistant and extremely drug-resistant strains of the bacillus (MDR-TB and XDR-TB, respectively) remains an ongoing concern.

Fungal Infections

Fungal infections, including histoplasmosis, coccidioidomycosis, and blastomycosis, can cause pneumonia. Because the organisms are endemic to particular regions of the country, infection is generally only seen in individuals who live in or travel to regions associated with these organisms, such as the San Joaquin Valley in California or other areas of the southwestern United States where coccidioidomycosis is seen. Many infections are asymptomatic while severe disease may be seen with large exposure or in immunocompromised individuals. *Cryptococcus* species can also cause pneumonia in both immunocompetent and immunosuppressed individuals.

Pulmonary Involvement in HIV

HIV frequently involves the lung, with the risk and type of infection being a function of the degree of immunosuppression. Bacterial pneumonia and tuberculosis may occur with any degree of immunosuppression while infections such as *Pneumocystis jirovecii, Mycobacterium avium-intracellulare*, and cytomegalovirus infections occur when the CD4+ count falls below certain thresholds. Kaposi's sarcoma may occur in the lung. When patients from high-risk groups, such as people who use injection drugs or engage in frequent unprotected intercourse, present with these pulmonary problems, they should be evaluated for HIV.

SUPPURATIVE DISEASES

Bronchiectasis

This disease is characterized by permanent dilatation of bronchi with local suppuration. It results from chronic infection and inflammation and, in some cases impaired airway clearance, and can be seen in conjunction with a variety of problems including recurrent pneumonia, immune deficiencies such as hypogammaglobulinemia, ciliary dyskinesias, or airway occlusion due to, for example, a retained airway foreign body or chronic extrinsic compression.

Pathology

The mucosal surface of the affected bronchi shows loss of ciliated epithelium, squamous metaplasia, and infiltration with inflammatory cells. Pus is present in the lumen during infective exacerbations. In advanced stages, the surrounding lung often shows fibrosis and chronic inflammatory changes.

Clinical Features

The cardinal feature is a chronic productive cough with copious amounts of yellow or green sputum that can be exacerbated following upper respiratory tract infections. Patients may have halitosis and are prone to massive hemoptysis due to hypertrophy of the bronchial circulation. Crepitations are often heard, and finger clubbing is seen in severe cases. The chest radiograph shows increased parenchymal markings and dilated airways with thickened walls. Dilated airways are readily seen on CT scans of the chest (Figure 7.10).

Pulmonary Function

Mild disease causes no loss of function. In more advanced cases, there is a reduction of FEV_1 and FVC because of chronic inflammatory changes, including fibrosis. Radioactive isotope measurements show reduced ventilation and pulmonary blood flow in the affected area, but there may be a greatly increased bronchial artery supply to the diseased tissue. Hypoxemia may develop as a result of blood flow through unventilated lung.

Cystic Fibrosis

Cystic fibrosis (CF) is caused by the loss of function of the cystic fibrosis transmembrane regulator (CFTR), a transmembrane protein present in a variety of cell types and tissues. While the lung is the primary affected organ, CF also affects the liver, pancreas, gonads, and other organs.

Pathogenesis

Although the ΔF508 mutation is the most common mutation, there are a large number of mutations that affect the CFTR. These manifest in a variety of ways including absent or defective production of the protein or abnormal

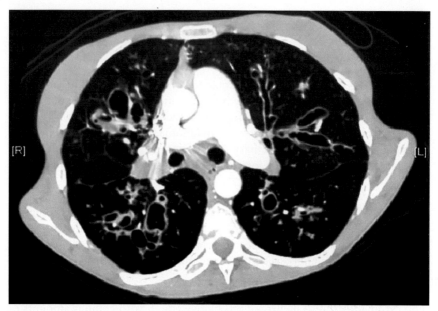

Figure 7.10. CT scan of the chest demonstrating dilated, thickened airways in a patient with bronchiectasis due to cystic fibrosis.

folding, regulation, or transport of the protein to the cell membrane. The net result of all of these defects are varying degrees of impaired sodium and chloride transport, which lead to impaired mucous clearance or plugging of airways or ducts. In the lungs, decreased sodium efflux from the respiratory epithelium reduces hydration of the periciliary mucous layer, which impairs mucociliary clearance and predisposes to infection. The airways inevitably become colonized with pathogenic bacteria, including *Staphylococcus aureus*, *Pseudomonas aeruginosa*, and *Burkholderia cepacia*.

Atrophy of pancreatic tissue and dilation of pancreatic ducts can occur, leading to both exocrine and endocrine insufficiency. The first impairs absorption of fat-soluble vitamins causing malnutrition, while the second leads to diabetes mellitus. Thickened secretions and chronic inflammation in the bile ductules can lead to portal hypertension and cirrhosis. The majority of male patients are infertile due to obstructive azoospermia from absence or atrophy of male reproductive tract structures.

Clinical Features

Some patients present with features of the disease at birth or early in life such as meconium ileus, recurrent infections, or slower than expected growth. Less severe presentations related to less common mutations might not occur until later in childhood or even adulthood. The respiratory symptoms include cough productive of copious thick sputum, frequent chest infections, and decreased exercise tolerance. Large-volume hemoptysis occurs in some patients due to bleeding from bronchiectatic airways supplied by a hypertrophied bronchial circulation. Finger clubbing is often prominent. Auscultation may reveal coarse rales and rhonchi. The chest radiograph is abnormal early in the disease and shows areas of consolidation, fibrosis, and cystic changes. Many cases are now detected with neonatal screening for elevated serum immunoreactive trypsinogen or DNA analysis for CFTR variants. Diagnosis is confirmed by finding elevated sweat chloride levels, specific gene mutations, or an abnormal nasal potential difference.

For many years, death almost invariably occurred before adulthood, but with improved treatment focused on secretion clearance, suppressive antibiotic therapy, aggressive treatment of exacerbations, and new classes of medications that target the specific molecular defects in CFTR, the median survival is now greater than 45 years of age.

Pulmonary Function

An abnormal distribution of ventilation and an increased alveolar–arterial P_{O_2} difference are early changes. Some investigators report that tests of small-airway function, such as flow rates at low lung volumes, may detect minimal disease. There are decreases in FEV_1 and $FEF_{25\%-75\%}$ that do not respond to bronchodilators. RV and FRC are raised and there may be loss of elastic recoil. Exercise tolerance falls as the disease progresses and in later stages patients often manifest a mixed obstructive–restrictive defect on pulmonary function testing.

KEY CONCEPTS

1. The most important atmospheric pollutants include carbon monoxide, oxides of nitrogen and sulfur, hydrocarbons, particulates, and photochemical oxidants.

2. Most pollutants occur as aerosols and are deposited in the lung by impaction, sedimentation, or diffusion.

3. Deposited pollutants are removed by the mucociliary system in the airways and macrophages in the alveoli.

4. Coal worker's pneumoconiosis and silicosis result from long-term exposure to coal dust and silica, respectively. In their mild forms, they cause dyspnea and cough together with micronodular lesions on chest radiography, while more severe disease leads to severe dyspnea and exercise limitation, more extensive radiographic opacities and, in some cases, progressive respiratory failure

5. Other pneumoconioses include asbestos-related diseases and berylliosis. Byssinosis caused by organic cotton dust and occupational asthma are examples of airway-centric diseases caused by inhaled organic dusts.

6. Infectious diseases of the lung including bacterial and viral pneumonia, fungal infections, and tuberculosis are an important source of morbidity and mortality in high- and low-income countries.

7. Bronchial carcinoma is largely caused by cigarette smoking and is the most common cause of cancer-related death in the United States. The prognosis varies based on the type and stage of the cancer.

8. Cystic fibrosis is caused by a genetic abnormality of the cystic fibrosis transmembrane regulator, which causes abnormal mucus, bronchiectasis, and impaired pulmonary function.

CLINICAL VIGNETTE

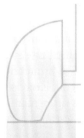

A 19-year-old man presents to the emergency department after coughing up a large amount of blood. During an evaluation by his pediatrician at the age of 5 for recurrent sinus and respiratory infections, he was found to have an elevated sweat chloride and two gene mutations associated with cystic fibrosis. He was on appropriate treatment for several years, but since dropping out of school and moving out of his parents' house, he has not been taking any medications or doing his regular airway clearance techniques. He states that his breathing has been getting worse over the past 6 months and that he has a daily cough productive of large amounts of thick yellow sputum. On examination, he is afebrile but tachypneic. He has diffuse rhonchi throughout his lungs, a prolonged expiratory phase, and finger clubbing. A chest radiograph is obtained and shows the following:

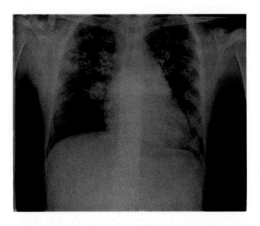

(Continued)

Questions

- What is the pathophysiological basis of his disease?
- What are the tubular structures seen in the mid-upper lung zones on his chest radiograph?
- What changes in pulmonary function would you expect to see on detailed pulmonary function testing?
- Why are regular airway clearance techniques important for the long-term health of this patient?
- Why is he coughing up large amounts of blood?

QUESTIONS

For each question, choose the one best answer.

1. A 70-year-old man with no smoking history presents with 8 months of worsening dyspnea and a nonproductive cough. He spent many years as an insulation worker in the shipyards. On exam, he has a fast respiratory rate with small volumes, and fine crepitations at the bases of his lungs. A plain chest radiograph reveals basilar net-like opacities and calcified pleural plaques. Spirometry shows an FEV_1 65% predicted, an FVC 69% predicted, and FEV_1/FVC 0.83. Which of the following is the most likely diagnosis?
   A. Asbestosis
   B. Berylliosis
   C. Chronic obstructive pulmonary disease
   D. Coal worker's pneumoconiosis
   E. Silicosis

2. A 24-year-old woman with a 5-year history of injection drug use but no other past medical history is evaluated for worsening dyspnea and a dry cough over a period of 2 weeks. On exam, she is tachypneic with an oxygen saturation of 85% breathing air. Her neck veins are not elevated, her cardiac exam is normal, and she has diffuse rhonchi on auscultation. After a chest radiograph reveals diffuse bilateral opacities, a sputum sample is obtained and shows evidence of *Pneumocystis jirovecii* pneumonia. Which of the following is the most appropriate next diagnostic test?
   A. Echocardiography
   B. HIV antibody test
   C. Spirometry
   D. Sweat chloride testing
   E. Tuberculosis skin test

3. An accident occurs in a local paper mill. As part of the emergency response, an environmental services engineer measures the size (noted by their diameter) and amount of the particles released into the factory space occupied by the workers at the time of the accident and derives the following frequency histogram.

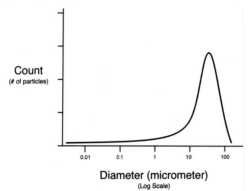

Where in the respiratory tracts of the workers in the plant at the time of the accident were the particles most likely to have deposited?
A. Alveolar space
B. Bronchi
C. Nose and nasopharynx
D. Respiratory bronchioles
E. Terminal bronchioles

4. A 46-year-old man is evaluated in the emergency department for 2 days of fever, worsening dyspnea, and cough productive of rust-colored sputum. His oxygen saturation at the time of presentation is 88% while breathing ambient air while his blood pressure is 115/78 mm Hg. His mental status is normal, but he is tachypneic, with dullness to percussion and decreased breath sounds at his right lung base. His skin is warm and not mottled. A chest radiograph demonstrates a focal opacity in the right lower lobe. Which of the following is the most likely cause of this patient's hypoxemia?
A. Decreased cardiac output
B. Diffusion impairment
C. Hypoventilation
D. Hypoxic vasoconstriction
E. Shunt

5. A 12-year-old girl is sent to the pediatric pulmonary clinic for evaluation of recurrent respiratory tract infections. Her mother notes that she has had multiple episodes of pneumonia and sinus infections in the past

10 years. Even between these infections she commonly has a cough productive of thick sputum. Her weight is in the 20th percentile for her age, and on exam she has scattered expiratory wheezes. A chest radiograph is performed and shows multiple dilated airways with thickened airway walls. Genetic testing is performed, and she is found to be a homozygote for the ΔF508 mutation. Which of the following defects in immune system or airway function most likely accounts for the observed problems in this patient?

A. Decreased complement activity
B. Decreased sodium efflux from the respiratory epithelium
C. Impaired B-cell function
D. Impaired neutrophil phagocytosis
E. Increased bronchial hyperreactivity

6. A 55-year-old construction worker presents to the emergency department following a work-related exposure to a poorly soluble, but potentially toxic gas. Which location in the respiratory tract would be the site of the greatest deposition of the gas molecules?

A. Nasal passages
B. Posterior oropharynx
C. Trachea
D. Mainstem bronchi
E. Respiratory bronchioles

7. A 51-year-old man is evaluated for worsening dyspnea on exertion and a chronic productive cough over a 9-month period. He is a former smoker and spent 30 years working as a sandblaster before retiring 2 years ago due to chronic back pain. On examination, he is mildly tachypneic and has scattered end-inspiratory crepitations on lung auscultation. Pulmonary function testing reveals an FEV_1/FVC ratio of 0.65, total lung capacity 68% predicted, and diffusing capacity for carbon monoxide of 55% predicted. A chest radiograph is performed and is shown below.

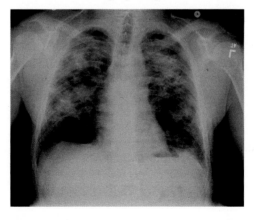

For which of the following is the patient at increased risk compared to healthy individuals?

A. Arteriovenous malformation
B. Legionellosis
C. Pneumococcal pneumonia
D. Venous thromboembolism
E. Tuberculosis

8. A 67-year-old woman with a 30-pack-year history of smoking presents for evaluation of hemoptysis. She reports coughing up coin-sized amounts of blood and notes worsening dyspnea on exertion and 5 kg weight loss in the past 2 months. A chest CT scan is performed and shows no evidence of lung opacities or emphysema but does reveal a possible mass in the right main bronchus. She is referred for bronchoscopy, which demonstrates an endobronchial lesion causing a 50% narrowing of the diameter of that airway. Which of the following would you expect to see on pulmonary function testing in this patient?

A. Decreased closing volume
B. Decreased FEV_1/FVC ratio
C. Decreased residual volume
D. Decreased total lung capacity
E. Increased diffusing capacity for carbon monoxide

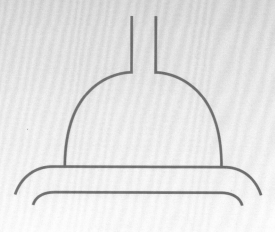

Part 3

Function of the
Failing Lung

Respiratory failure is the result of many types of acute or chronic lung disease. Part three is devoted to the physiologic principles of respiratory failure and its chief modes of treatment: oxygen administration and mechanical ventilation.

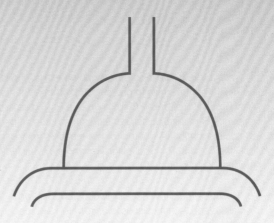

Respiratory Failure

8

Respiratory failure is said to occur when the lung fails to oxygenate the arterial blood adequately and/or fails to prevent CO_2 retention. It can be an acute or chronic process. Although a P_{O_2} of below 60 mm Hg or a P_{CO_2} greater than 50 mm Hg are often cited as evidence of respiratory failure, there are no absolute thresholds for these values. Instead, the determination of whether or not a patient is in respiratory failure depends on not only the P_{O_2} and P_{CO_2} but also a variety of clinical factors. At the end of this chapter, the reader should be able to:

- Describe the differences between acute, chronic, and acute on chronic respiratory failure and identify diseases associated with each entity
- Describe the causes and effects of hypoxemia and hypercapnia in patients with respiratory failure
- Describe the pulmonary function abnormalities in respiratory failure including changes in acid–base status, resistance, compliance, and neuromuscular function
- Describe the pathological and clinical features and pulmonary function abnormalities in the acute and neonatal respiratory distress syndromes
- Outline the basic treatment principles for respiratory failure and how they relate to abnormalities in pulmonary function

TYPES OF RESPIRATORY FAILURE

Respiratory failure is a broad term that encompasses many entities. These can be grouped into one of three general categories.

Acute Respiratory Failure

This category includes processes that progress to respiratory failure over a short period of time lasting from just a few minutes to several days. Examples include infections such as severe viral or bacterial pneumonias, asthma exacerbations, pulmonary embolism, and exposure to inhaled toxic substances such as chlorine gas or oxides of nitrogen. While many cases of acute respiratory failure are primarily problems of oxygenation (acute hypoxemic respiratory failure), other acute processes are primarily disorders of impaired ventilation (acute hypercarbic respiratory failure) such as occurs following an opiate overdose or with acute neuromuscular disorders such as Guillain-Barré syndrome or botulism.

Chronic Respiratory Failure

This category includes diseases in which problems with oxygenation and/or ventilation persist for months to years. The best examples include those individuals with chronic hypoxemia and/or CO_2 retention due to severe chronic obstructive pulmonary disease (COPD) and those with chronic hypoxemic respiratory failure due to idiopathic pulmonary fibrosis. The latter group may develop chronic ventilatory failure in the advanced stages of their disease. Chronic ventilatory failure can also be seen in individuals with severe morbid obesity as well as those with chronic neuromuscular conditions such as Duchenne muscular dystrophy, postpolio syndrome, and amyotrophic lateral sclerosis. Such patients are usually capable of limited physical activity despite the chronically low P_{O_2} and elevated P_{CO_2}.

Acute on Chronic Respiratory Failure

This refers to an acute worsening of symptoms and pulmonary function in those with long-standing cardiopulmonary disease. It is an important and common problem in individuals with COPD, cystic fibrosis, heart failure, and idiopathic pulmonary fibrosis. Under usual conditions, these patients live in a state of either stable or slowly declining lung function and have limited physiologic reserve. In response to respiratory tract infections or other inciting events that are not always identified, they can experience marked worsening of ventilation–perfusion relationships or lung mechanics, which due to the limited reserves of pulmonary function, rapidly worsen hypoxemia, ventilation, and/or the work of breathing.

PULMONARY FUNCTION IN RESPIRATORY FAILURE

Various changes in pulmonary function can be seen in individuals with respiratory failure, with the particular mix and magnitude of changes varying from person to person based on the cause of respiratory failure and the rapidity of onset.

Hypoxemia

Hypoxemia is a common feature of most forms of respiratory failure. While signs such as cyanosis, tachycardia, and altered mental status provide clues to its presence, most patients are initially identified as being hypoxemic by the finding of a low oxygen saturation on pulse oximetry. Once hypoxemia is identified in this way, measuring the P_{O_2} by arterial blood gas is helpful to determine the degree of hypoxemia and assess the underlying cause.

Causes of Hypoxemia

Any of the four mechanisms of hypoxemia—hypoventilation, diffusion impairment, shunt, and ventilation–perfusion inequality—can contribute to the severe hypoxemia of respiratory failure. However, the most important cause by far is ventilation–perfusion inequality (including blood flow through unventilated lung). This mechanism is largely responsible for the low arterial P_{O_2} in respiratory failure complicating obstructive diseases, restrictive diseases, pulmonary vascular diseases, and the acute respiratory distress syndrome (ARDS).

Effects of Hypoxemia

Mild hypoxemia produces few physiologic changes. It should be recalled that the arterial oxygen saturation is still approximately 90% when the P_{O_2} is only 60 mm Hg at a normal pH (see Figure 2.1). The only abnormalities are a slight impairment of mental performance, diminished visual acuity, and perhaps mild hyperventilation.

When the arterial P_{O_2} drops quickly below 40 to 50 mm Hg, deleterious effects can be seen in several organ systems with the extent of the problems varying based on the age and underlying health status of the affected individual. The central nervous system is particularly vulnerable, and the patient often has headache, somnolence, or altered mental status. Profound acute hypoxemia may cause convulsions, retinal hemorrhages, and ischemic brain injury. Tachycardia and mild hypertension are often seen, partly due to the release of catecholamines, but in severe cases, patients can develop bradycardia and hypotension and even go into cardiac arrest. Renal function is impaired, and sodium retention and proteinuria may be seen. Pulmonary hypertension can also be seen.

Tissue Hypoxia

While the arterial P_{O_2} is an important concern in respiratory failure, the more important issue is whether oxygen delivery to the tissues is sufficient to satisfy metabolic needs and avoid tissue hypoxia. In addition to the P_{O_2}, oxygen delivery is a function of multiple factors, including the oxygen capacity of the blood, the oxygen affinity of the hemoglobin, cardiac output, and the distribution of blood flow. Individuals with a low P_{O_2} can still maintain adequate oxygen delivery and avoid tissue hypoxia if they have a normal cardiac function and hemoglobin concentration. Similarly, tissue hypoxia can develop even when the arterial P_{O_2} is normal if there is severe impairment of cardiac function or the individual has suffered significant blood loss.

Tissues vary considerably in their vulnerability to hypoxia. Those at greatest risk include the central nervous system and the myocardium. Cessation of blood flow to the cerebral cortex results in loss of function within 4 to 6 seconds, loss of consciousness in 10 to 20 seconds, and irreversible changes in 3 to 5 minutes.

If the tissue P_{O_2} falls below a critical level, aerobic oxidation ceases and anaerobic glycolysis takes over with the formation and release of increasing amounts of lactic acid. The P_{O_2} at which this occurs is not accurately known and probably varies among tissues. However, there is evidence that the critical intracellular P_{O_2} is of the order of 1 to 3 mm Hg in the region of the mitochondria. Anaerobic glycolysis is a relatively inefficient method of obtaining energy from glucose. Nevertheless, it plays a critical role in maintaining tissue viability in respiratory failure. Large amounts of lactic acid are formed and released into the blood, causing a metabolic acidosis. If tissue oxygenation subsequently improves, the lactic acid can be reconverted to glucose or used directly for energy. Most of this reconversion takes place in the liver.

Hypercapnia

Causes of Hypercapnia

CO_2 retention can develop in respiratory failure as a result of hypoventilation and ventilation–perfusion inequality. Hypoventilation is the cause in respiratory failure resulting from neuromuscular diseases such as amyotrophic lateral sclerosis, botulism, Guillain-Barré syndrome, and poliomyelitis or from opiate overdoses and chest wall abnormalities such as severe kyphoscoliosis (see Figure 2.3 and Table 2.1). Ventilation–perfusion inequality is the culprit in severe COPD and long-standing diffuse parenchymal lung disease. Despite the presence of severe ventilation–perfusion abnormality, some patients still have a normal or low arterial P_{CO_2} due to increases in ventilation, which facilitates elimination of CO_2.

An important cause of worsening hypercarbia in some patients with respiratory failure is the injudicious use of oxygen therapy. This can occur for two reasons. First, many patients with severe COPD have chronic CO_2 retention and hypoxemia. While the ventilatory responses to CO_2 are blunted in these individuals due to compensatory acid–base changes in the blood and CSF, hypoxemia provides an added stimulus to ventilation above their basal respiratory drive. Application of excessive supplemental oxygen and overly large increases in the arterial P_{O_2} abolish the hypoxic ventilatory response, leading to a fall in minute ventilation. Second, by raising the alveolar P_{O_2} with supplemental oxygen, there is release of hypoxic vasoconstriction in poorly ventilated areas of lung. This, in turn, causes increased blood flow to the poorly ventilated areas, which worsens ventilation–perfusion inequality and promotes CO_2 retention. This process of worsening hypercarbia with supplemental oxygen administration can also be seen in individuals with the obesity hypoventilation syndrome.

Effects of Hypercapnia

Increased P_{CO_2} has multiple effects including increased cerebral blood flow and intracranial pressure, increased central and peripheral chemoreceptor stimulation, enhanced hypoxic pulmonary vasoconstriction, bronchodilation in the distal airways, and a rightward shift in the hemoglobin–oxygen dissociation curve (Bohr effect). One of the most important effects from a clinical standpoint is altered mental status in response to severe acute hypercapnia, a phenomenon sometimes referred to as CO_2 narcosis. Respiratory drive and minute ventilation initially rise following increases in arterial P_{CO_2}, but if these responses fail to correct the problem and the P_{CO_2} rises further, the individual may develop a depressed level of consciousness. Other clinical effects include restlessness, tremor, slurred speech, asterixis (flapping tremor), and fluctuations of mood.

Acid–Base

Because the various forms of respiratory failure occur over varying time frames and are associated with different degrees of hypoxemia and CO_2 retention, a variety of acid–base abnormalities can be seen. To appreciate these changes, we can begin by examining Figure 8.1, which shows an O_2–CO_2 diagram (see *West's Respiratory Physiology: The Essentials*, 11th ed., pp. 199-202) with the line for a respiratory exchange ratio of 0.8.

Pure *hypoventilation* leading to respiratory failure moves the arterial P_{O_2} and P_{CO_2} in the direction indicated by arrow A. In these situations, the alveolar–arterial P_{O_2} difference is normal. If this is an acute change, as can be seen with an opiate overdose or in the early phases of Guillain-Barré syndrome (see Figures 2.2 and 2.3), an arterial blood gas will demonstrate an acute respiratory acidosis. If hypoventilation persists for several days or more, as seen with muscular dystrophy, for example, renal compensation will raise the serum bicarbonate, which increases the arterial pH toward normal. This pattern is referred to as a compensated respiratory acidosis.

Severe *ventilation–perfusion ratio inequality* is associated with an increased alveolar–arterial P_{O_2} difference. Most cases are associated with movement along either lines C or D. Provided there is no tissue hypoxia and lactic acidosis, the former is not associated with changes in acid–base status because the P_{CO_2} is unchanged while the latter causes a respiratory alkalosis. Acute problems such as pneumonia or ARDS cause an acute respiratory alkalosis, while more chronic problems such as idiopathic pulmonary fibrosis are marked by compensatory changes in serum bicarbonate and a decrease in arterial pH toward normal. When alveolar ventilation is inadequate to maintain a normal arterial P_{CO_2}, movement occurs along line B. This pattern is frequently seen in very severe COPD or very advanced stages of idiopathic pulmonary fibrosis. In such cases, patients manifest a compensated respiratory acidosis.

As noted above, patients with severe chronic lung disease and a compensated respiratory acidosis sometimes develop an exacerbation of their disease, leading to a further increase in the P_{CO_2} above the typical baseline.

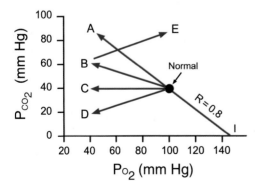

Figure 8-1. Patterns of arterial P_{O_2} and P_{CO_2} in different types of respiratory failure. Note that the P_{CO_2} can be high, as in pure hypoventilation (*line A*), or low, as in ARDS (*line D*). (See text for further details.)

This will cause the pH to fall below normal until sufficient time elapses for additional renal compensation. Administration of excessive supplemental oxygen to a patient with COPD and CO_2 retention will improve the P_{O_2} but, as noted above, may increase P_{CO_2} due to decreased ventilation and changes in ventilation–perfusion matching due to reduction of hypoxic pulmonary vasoconstriction. This corresponds to a move from B to E in Figure 8.1 and would be associated with worsening acidemia.

The acidemia seen in many cases of respiratory failure may also worsen if CO_2 retention is accompanied by severe hypoxemia and tissue hypoxia, which, as noted, can lead to liberation of lactic acid and a metabolic acidosis. This can be exacerbated by factors that impair end-organ perfusion such as shock or decreased venous return due to increased intrathoracic pressure during mechanical ventilation.

Airway Resistance

In patients with COPD and asthma, respiratory failure is often precipitated by an increase in airway resistance. This can occur due to a combination of increased secretions and bronchospasm following a viral respiratory tract infection or exposure to smog or cold air. Increased airway resistance also plays a prominent role in patients with pulmonary edema due to a combination of edema fluid in the airways, reflex bronchoconstriction due to stimulation of irritant receptors in the airway walls, and peribronchial cuffing from interstitial edema (see Figure 6.5).

Compliance

Problems involving the lung parenchyma as well as the abdomen, chest wall, and pleural space can reduce the compliance of the respiratory system. Such changes can occur acutely, as happens with pulmonary edema and ARDS, or develop more chronically, as in idiopathic pulmonary fibrosis. When this occurs, a greater change in pressure is required to achieve a given tidal volume and maintain adequate ventilation. This requires a higher work of breathing, which can be difficult to sustain depending on the severity of the problem and the individual's underlying cardiopulmonary reserve. Decreases in tidal volume can be compensated for by increasing the respiratory rate, but the work of breathing is still increased due to increased ventilation requirements resulting from the higher dead space fraction.

Neuromuscular Function

Changes in neuromuscular function can be both a cause and a consequence of respiratory failure. From a causal perspective, respiratory failure may occur when brainstem respiratory centers are depressed by drugs, such as opiates and benzodiazepines or with problems affecting peripheral nerves, as in amyotrophic lateral sclerosis and Guillain-Barré syndrome, the neuromuscular junction as in myasthenia gravis, and anticholinesterase poisoning or the muscles themselves, as in muscular dystrophy (see Figure 2.3 and Table 2.1). Abnormalities of the chest wall, as occurs in kyphoscoliosis or severe flail chest following chest trauma, can also cause respiratory failure.

Diaphragm Fatigue

In addition to these primary neuromuscular problems, fatigue of the diaphragm is another contributor to the hypoventilation of respiratory failure. Fatigue can be defined as a loss of contractile force after work; it can be measured directly from the transdiaphragmatic pressure resulting from a maximum contraction or indirectly from the muscle relaxation time or the electromyogram, although neither technique is commonly used at the bedside. The diaphragm consists of striated skeletal muscle innervated by the phrenic nerves. Although the diaphragm is predominantly made up of slow-twitch oxidative fibers and fast-twitch oxidative glycolytic fibers, which are relatively resistant to fatigue, this can occur if the work of breathing is greatly increased over prolonged periods of time. Infants have fewer fatigue-resistant fibers compared to adults, which predisposes to more rapid onset of respiratory failure in the setting of acute respiratory disease.

There is evidence that some patients with severe COPD continually breathe close to the work level at which fatigue occurs and that an exacerbation or infection can tip them into a fatigue state. This will then result in hypoventilation, CO_2 retention, and severe hypoxemia. Because hypercapnia impairs diaphragm contractility and severe hypoxemia accelerates the onset of fatigue, a vicious cycle develops. This situation can be limited by reducing the work of breathing by treating bronchospasm and controlling infection, and by giving oxygen judiciously to relieve the hypoxemia. While the administration of methylxanthines may improve diaphragm contractility and also relieve reversible bronchoconstriction, they are no longer widely used in clinical practice. Over the long-term, the force of contraction can be improved through pulmonary rehabilitation programs.

Acquired Weakness

Patients with respiratory failure who require invasive mechanical ventilation over many days to weeks can develop polyneuropathy and/or myopathy, which lead(s) to weakness of the diaphragm and other muscles of respiration. The precise mechanism for this problem, often referred to as ICU-acquired weakness, is not clear but may relate to an enhanced catabolic state in critical illness, structural muscle alterations, microcirculatory changes, mitochondrial dysfunction, and nerve and muscle membrane ion channel dysfunction. As a result, even though the primary problem that led to respiratory failure may resolve, the affected individuals may be unable to sustain adequate ventilation on their own and have difficulty surviving without the mechanical ventilator.

RESPIRATORY DISTRESS SYNDROMES

There are two forms of severe acute hypoxemic respiratory failure that warrant special attention, one seen in children, adolescents, and adults following various types of insults and another seen specifically in neonates following premature birth.

Acute Respiratory Distress Syndrome

Formerly known as adult respiratory distress syndrome (ARDS) occurs as the end result of a variety of injuries that are either intrinsic to the lung, such as pneumonia or aspiration, or extrinsic to the lung such as trauma, burns, nonpulmonary sepsis, and pancreatitis.

Pathology

The early changes consist of interstitial and alveolar edema. Hemorrhage, cellular debris, and proteinaceous fluid are present in the alveoli; hyaline membranes (Figure 8.2) may be seen; and there is patchy atelectasis. Later, hyperplasia and organization occur. The damaged alveolar epithelium becomes lined with type 2 alveolar epithelial cells, and there is cellular infiltration of the alveolar walls. Eventually, interstitial fibrosis may develop, although complete healing can occur.

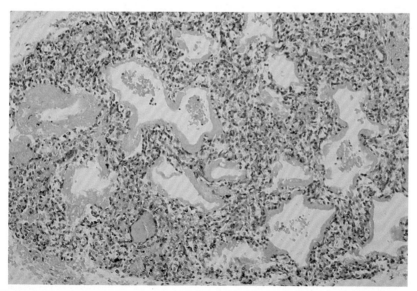

Figure 8.2. Histologic changes in ARDS as found on autopsy. There are patchy atelectasis, edema, hyaline membranes, and hemorrhage in the alveoli as well as inflammatory cells in the alveolar walls. (Image courtesy of Edward Klatt, MD.)

Pathogenesis

This is still unclear and many factors may play a role. As a result of the initial injury, proinflammatory cytokines including various interleukins and tumor necrosis factor are released, leading to neutrophil recruitment and activation. These neutrophils subsequently release reactive oxygen species, proteases, and cytokines that damage type I alveolar epithelial cells and capillary endothelial cells. This leads to impaired surfactant function and increased capillary permeability, which, in turn, cause atelectasis and flooding of the alveoli and interstitium with proteinaceous fluid.

Clinical Features

ARDS may develop anywhere from several hours to 7 days following the initial insult. The onset is typically heralded by worsening hypoxemia and increasing oxygen requirements, at which time the chest radiograph typically shows bilateral alveolar opacities as in Figure 8.3. Patients typically have markedly increased work of breathing due to the severe hypoxemia and reduced compliance, and diffuse crepitations on lung examination. Invasive mechanical

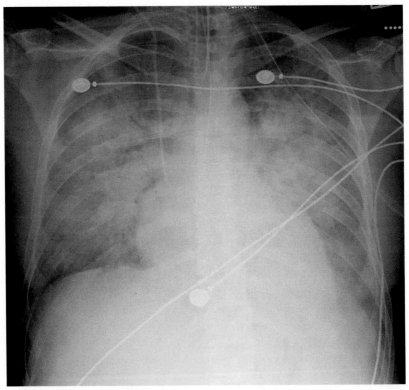

Figure 8.3. Plain chest radiograph showing typical bilateral alveolar opacities in the acute respiratory distress syndrome.

ventilation is frequently necessary to support oxygenation and ventilation, although select patients can be managed with noninvasive means. While the severity of hypoxemia can be assessed by measuring the alveolar–arterial P_{O_2} difference, in clinical practice, this is commonly done by calculating the ratio of the arterial P_{O_2} and the inspired oxygen fraction, referred to as the Pa_{O_2}/F_IO_2 or P/F ratio. The diagnosis of ARDS requires a P/F ratio below 300. The lower the value, the worse the ventilation–perfusion inequality.

Pulmonary Function

The lung becomes very stiff, and unusually high distending pressures are required to inflate them. Associated with this reduced compliance is a marked fall in FRC. The cause of the increased recoil is presumably the alveolar edema and exudate that exaggerate the surface tension forces. As was pointed out in Chapter 6 (see Figure 6.3), edematous alveoli have a reduced volume. Interstitial edema also contributes to the abnormal stiffness of the lungs.

Acute Respiratory Distress Syndrome (ARDS)

- End result of a variety of insults including trauma and infection
- Alveolar edema and exudate with opacification on the radiograph
- Severe hypoxemia
- Low lung compliance
- Mechanical ventilation typically required

As would be expected from the histologic and radiologic appearances of the lung (Figures 8.2 and 8.3), there is marked ventilation–perfusion inequality, with a substantial fraction of the total blood flow going to unventilated alveoli. This fraction may reach 50% or more. Figure 8.4 shows some results obtained by the multiple inert gas method in a 44-year-old patient who developed respiratory failure after an automobile accident and who was mechanically ventilated. Note the presence of blood flow to lung units with abnormally low ventilation–perfusion ratios and also the shunt of 8% (compare the normal distribution in Figure 2.9). Figure 8.4 also shows a large amount of ventilation going to units with high ventilation–perfusion ratios. One reason for this is the abnormally high airway pressures developed by the ventilator, which reduce the blood flow in some alveoli (compare Figure 10.4).

The ventilation–perfusion inequality and shunt cause profound hypoxemia, which can only be corrected with high inspired oxygen concentrations and increased positive end-expiratory pressure (discussed in Chapter 10). In very severe cases, other interventions including inhaled pulmonary vasodilators, ventilation in the prone position, neuromuscular blockade, and extracorporeal membrane oxygenation may be used to maintain an adequate arterial P_{O_2}.

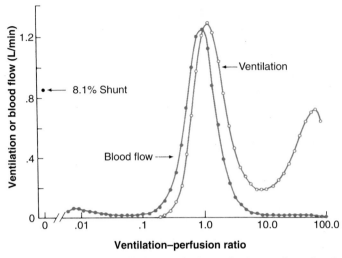

Figure 8.4. Distribution of ventilation–perfusion ratios in a patient who developed ARDS after a motor vehicle collision. Note the 8% shunt and the blood flow to units with low ventilation–perfusion ratios. In addition, there is some ventilation to high $\dot{V}_A/\dot{Q}$ units, probably as a result of the high airway pressure developed by the ventilator (compare Figure 10-4).

The arterial P_{CO_2} varies significantly between patients. Some patients have a low or normal P_{CO_2} despite the severe ventilation–perfusion inequality and shunt while others develop hypercarbia due to a significant increase in the physiologic dead space.

Neonatal Respiratory Distress Syndrome

This condition, which has also been called hyaline membrane disease of the newborn and infant respiratory distress syndrome, has several features in common with ARDS. Pathologically, the lung shows hemorrhagic edema, patchy atelectasis, and hyaline membranes caused by proteinaceous fluid and cellular debris within the alveoli. Physiologically, there is profound hypoxemia, with both ventilation–perfusion inequality and blood flow through unventilated lung. A right-to-left shunt via the patent foramen ovale sometimes exaggerates the hypoxemia. Chest radiography typically shows diffuse bilateral alveolar opacities (Figure 8.5).

The chief cause of this condition is the absence of pulmonary surfactant. Surfactant is normally produced by the type 2 alveolar epithelial cells (see Figure 5.2) starting around the 20th week of gestation, although sufficient quantities are not present until much later in pregnancy. Infants born prematurely not only have insufficient quantities of surfactant but also impaired surfactant function due to differences in lipid and protein composition compared to surfactant in term infants. The ability of the infant to secrete surfactant

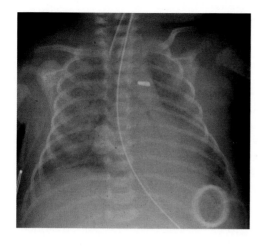

Figure 8-5. Radiograph showing typical changes of neonatal respiratory distress syndrome in a prematurely born infant. (Image courtesy of Jeffrey Otjen, MD.)

can be estimated by measuring the lecithin/sphingomyelin ratio of amniotic fluid. Maturation of the surfactant-synthesizing system can be hastened by the administration of corticosteroids to pregnant women anticipated to deliver at less than 34 weeks of gestation.

Treatment includes administration of exogenous surfactant as well as either nasal continuous positive airway pressure or invasive mechanical ventilation depending on the severity of the problem. High inspired oxygen concentrations and PEEP are often employed as well. Due to disruptions in the later stages of lung development, some survivors of neonatal respiratory distress syndrome develop bronchopulmonary dysplasia, a chronic lung disease marked by decreases in the size and number of alveoli and a persistent requirement for supplemental oxygen.

MANAGEMENT OF ACUTE RESPIRATORY FAILURE

There are two primary components to the management of acute respiratory failure: (1) treatment of the underlying problem by, for example, giving antibiotics to a patient with pneumonia or placing a tube in the intrapleural space (tube thoracostomy) in a patient with a large pneumothorax; and (2) correction of the deficits in pulmonary function. The first component varies significantly between disease processes and has been addressed in the discussions of various diseases in earlier chapters. The second component is considered in further detail below.

Hypoxemia

Hypoxemia is addressed by administering supplemental oxygen through a variety of invasive and noninvasive means described in detail in Chapters 9 and 10. The appropriate method and, in particular, the decision when to initiate invasive mechanical ventilation vary based on the severity of the patient's illness.

Hypercapnia

While patients with hypoventilation due to an opiate overdose can be readily treated with reversal agents like naloxone, most patients with acute or worsening hypercapnia require mechanical ventilatory support. This can be delivered either noninvasively through a tight-fitting mask or invasively through an endotracheal tube. These interventions are discussed in detail in Chapter 10.

Airway Resistance

When airway resistance is high due to increased airway secretions, treatment is directed at enhancing airway clearance. Because retained secretions are best removed by coughing, sustained work with respiratory therapists, nurses, and physicians on coughing and deep breathing exercises can be helpful. Maintenance of adequate hydration and humidification of supplemental oxygen prevents secretions from becoming too viscid and aids in clearance. While drugs such as aerosolized N-acetylcysteine to liquefy sputum are of little value in most patients, nebulized hypertonic saline and inhaled DNAase are useful in patients with bronchiectasis. Chest physiotherapy and postural drainage are helpful in select patients, while patients with impaired cough due to neuromuscular weakness benefit from use of mechanical insufflation–exsufflation devices.

Bronchoconstriction is addressed by administration of inhaled bronchodilators including albuterol and ipratropium. Corticosteroids are also given in asthma and COPD exacerbations to reduce underlying inflammation that contributes to the airway pathology. Finally, diuretics can be used to alleviate interstitial edema and peribronchial cuffing that contributes to increased resistance in some patients with exacerbations of heart failure.

Compliance

As noted earlier, compliance may be reduced due to problems involving the lung parenchyma, chest wall, pleural space, and abdomen. In some cases, such as severe pneumonia or ARDS, compliance only improves as the disease itself improves. In other cases, such as a patient with pulmonary edema and/or large pleural effusions, interventions such as diuresis or thoracentesis can lead to more rapid improvements in compliance and subsequent decreases in the work of breathing. Drainage of significant ascites or bowel decompression in a patient with severe ileus is sometimes used to address compliance problems related to abdominal distention.

Oxygen Delivery

In the face of hypoxemia, tissue oxygen delivery depends heavily on cardiac function and oxygen-carrying capacity. For this reason, support of the patient with respiratory failure sometimes requires interventions to support cardiac function or improve the hemoglobin concentration. Impaired cardiac function can be addressed through a variety of means, including inotropes such as dobutamine, diuretics, and mechanical circulatory support devices. Pulmonary vasodilators can decrease pulmonary artery pressure and improve right heart function in patients with pulmonary arterial hypertension but should be avoided in patients with pulmonary hypertension secondary to parenchymal lung diseases, such as COPD and idiopathic pulmonary fibrosis, due to a risk of worsening ventilation–perfusion matching. Patients who have a low stroke volume due to intravascular volume depletion benefit from fluid administration while those who are anemic may require red blood cell transfusion.

KEY CONCEPTS

1. Respiratory failure refers to the condition when the lung fails to oxygenate the blood adequately or fails to prevent CO_2 retention.

2. Hypoxemia is caused by hypoventilation, diffusion impairment, shunt, and ventilation–perfusion inequality, while CO_2 retention is due to hypoventilation and ventilation–perfusion inequality.

3. Severe hypoxemia causes many abnormalities including altered mental status, tachycardia, lactic acidosis, and proteinuria. CO_2 retention increases cerebral blood flow and may result in headache, confusion, or a decreased level of consciousness.

4. Acid–base and gas exchange abnormalities in respiratory failure vary depending on the causative disease and the chronicity of the problem.

5. The acute respiratory distress syndrome and neonatal respiratory distress syndrome are forms of severe respiratory failure characterized by severe hypoxemia, low lung compliance, and hyaline membranes on lung histology.

6. Management of respiratory failure involves treating the underlying cause and addressing the underlying deficits in pulmonary function by supporting oxygenation and ventilation, decreasing airway resistance, and improving compliance and oxygen delivery.

CLINICAL VIGNETTE

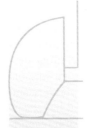

A 38-year-old woman with a history of chronic heavy alcohol use is admitted to the ICU with necrotizing pancreatitis. At the time of admission, she has an oxygen saturation of 97% breathing ambient air, a blood pressure of 89/67 mm Hg, and a chest radiograph without focal opacities. Following admission, she receives several liters of fluid to maintain an adequate mean arterial pressure. Four hours later, she complains of dyspnea and her oxygen saturation is noted to be only 90% while breathing ambient air. Despite starting her on oxygen by nasal cannula, her oxygen saturation continues to decrease and she develops increased dyspnea. Due to her worsening clinical condition, she is intubated and started on invasive mechanical ventilation. A chest radiograph performed following intubation shows diffuse bilateral opacities (shown below). An echocardiogram shows normal left ventricular function. An arterial blood gas is performed while she is receiving 100% oxygen and shows a pH of 7.45, P_{CO_2} of 35 mm Hg, P_{O_2} 66 of mm Hg, and HCO_3^- of 22 mmol/L.

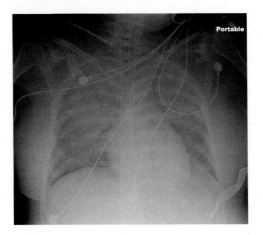

Questions

- Compared to the time of admission, what changes would you expect to see in her respiratory system compliance?
- What changes would you expect to see in her functional residual capacity?
- What is the most likely cause of her hypoxemia?
- Why is her arterial P_{CO_2} low despite the severity of her respiratory failure?

QUESTIONS

For each question, choose the one best answer.

1. A 71-year-old man presents to the Emergency Department with an exacerbation of his known severe chronic obstructive pulmonary disease with CO_2 retention. Following arrival, he is placed on oxygen by high-flow nasal cannula with an F_IO_2 of 1.0. His arterial blood gases before and after this intervention are shown in the table below.

F_IO_2	Arterial P_{O_2} (mm Hg)	Arterial P_{CO_2} (mm Hg)
0.21	50	50
1.0	450	80

Which of the following is the most likely cause for the observed change in P_{CO_2}?
A. Bohr effect
B. Decreased cardiac output
C. Decreased hypoxic pulmonary vasoconstriction
D. Increased airway resistance
E. Reduced 2,3-diphosphoglycerate concentration

2. A 58-year-old woman with severe COPD due to long-standing tobacco use presents to the Emergency Department with worsening dyspnea and headache during a chest infection. On examination, she is confused and restless and has a flapping tremor and diffuse expiratory wheezes. Which of the following would you most likely see on an arterial blood gas in this patient at the time she presents for evaluation?
A. High pH with a primary metabolic alkalosis
B. High pH with a primary respiratory alkalosis
C. Low pH with a primary metabolic acidosis
D. Low pH with a primary respiratory acidosis
E. Normal acid–base status

3. One day following admission for injuries suffered in a motorcycle collision, a 41-year-old man develops worsening hypoxemia. He is intubated and started on invasive mechanical ventilation during which time he has a Pa_{O_2}/F_IO_2 ratio of 105. A chest radiograph performed following intubation reveals diffuse bilateral opacities, while an echocardiogram demonstrates normal left ventricular systolic function. Which of the following changes in pulmonary function is most likely in this patient?

A. Decreased lung elastic recoil
B. Increased airway resistance
C. Increased blood flow to low $\dot{V}_A/\dot{Q}$ alveoli
D. Increased functional residual capacity
E. Increased lung compliance

4. Shortly after birth at only 31 weeks of gestation, a baby girl is noted to have nasal flaring, intercostal retractions, and hypoxemia on pulse oximetry. After a chest radiograph shows bilateral alveolar opacities, she is started on nasal continuous positive airway pressure. Which of the following medications should be also administered to speed resolution of her respiratory failure?
A. Digoxin
B. Furosemide
C. Inhaled albuterol
D. Inhaled ipratropium
E. Inhaled surfactant

5. A 62-year-old man with very severe COPD ($FEV_1 \sim 28\%$ predicted) presents with increasing cough, dyspnea, and sputum production following a viral upper respiratory infection. On examination, his S_pO_2 is 81% breathing ambient air, and he has a prolonged expiratory phase and diffuse musical sounds on expiration. Which of the following physiologic changes would you expect to see in his current clinical situation?
A. Decreased airway resistance
B. Decreased alveolar–arterial P_{O_2} difference
C. Decreased arterial P_{CO_2}
D. Increased arterial pH
E. Increased ventilation–perfusion mismatch

6. A 69-year-old woman presents to the hospital with 2 days of worsening dyspnea and is found to have an oxygen saturation of 81% breathing air. She is afebrile and confused and demonstrates accessory muscle use, bilateral crepitations on lung examination, a laterally displaced point of maximal cardiac impulse, pitting lower extremity edema, and cool, mottled distal extremities. Laboratory studies demonstrate a white blood cell count of 9×10^3 cells/μL (normal: 4 to 10 cells/μL), hemoglobin concentration of 12.8 g/dL (normal: 13 to 15 g/dL), lactate of 4.5 mmol/L (normal: less than 2 mmol/L), and arterial P_{CO_2} of 33 mm Hg. An echocardiogram shows a dilated, hypokinetic left ventricle with an ejection fraction of 41%. A chest radiograph is shown below.

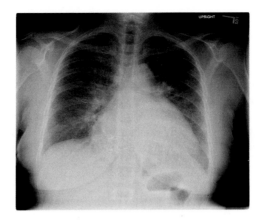

In addition to supplemental oxygen, which of the following interventions is indicated for treatment of this patient's respiratory failure?
A. Antibiotics
B. Dobutamine infusion
C. Inhaled surfactant
D. Noninvasive positive pressure ventilation
E. Red blood cell transfusion

7. A 32-year-old man is found unresponsive at home with an empty bottle of morphine at his side. He is brought into the Emergency Department where he is taking shallow breaths at a rate of 6 breaths per minute and has an oxygen saturation of 85% breathing air. A chest radiograph shows no focal opacities, cardiomegaly, or effusions. An arterial blood gas is obtained while he is breathing air and is shown in the table below:

pH	Arterial P_{CO_2} (mm Hg)	Arterial P_{O_2} (mm Hg)	Bicarbonate (mEq/L)
7.20	67	56	26

Which of the following is(are) the primary cause(s) of his hypoxemia?
A. Diffusion impairment
B. Hypoventilation
C. Shunt
D. Ventilation–perfusion inequality
E. Hypoventilation and perfusion inequality

8. A 39-year-old woman presents to the Emergency Department with 3 days of worsening fever, dyspnea, and productive cough. On examination, she has an oxygen saturation of 82% breathing air, dullness to percussion and decreased breath sounds at her right base. Her laboratory studies reveal an elevated white blood cell count and her chest radiograph demonstrates a focal opacity in the right middle and lower lobe without effusions or cardiomegaly. The figure below shows an O_2–CO_2 diagram for an individual at sea level with a respiratory exchange ratio of 0.8. To which of the points (A–E) would you expect this patient to move from the normal point as a result of her clinical presentation.

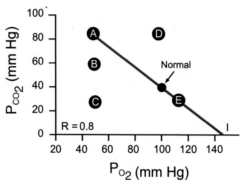

A. A
B. B
C. C
D. D
E. E

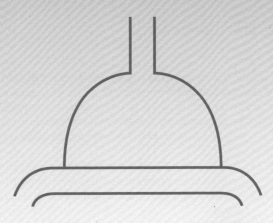

Oxygen Therapy

9

Oxygen administration has a critical role in the treatment of hypoxemia and especially in the management of respiratory failure. However, patients vary considerably in their response to oxygen, and several potential hazards are associated with its use. A clear understanding of the physiologic principles involved is necessary to maximize its utility and minimize complications. At the end of this chapter, the reader should be able to:

- Describe the relationship between the underlying cause of hypoxemia and the response to supplemental oxygen administration
- Identify factors that affect oxygen delivery and the oxygen content of mixed venous blood
- Describe the primary methods of supplemental oxygen administration
- Explain the mechanism by which excess supplemental oxygen administration may worsen CO_2 retention
- Describe the effect of oxygen administration on lung units with low ventilation–perfusion ratios

IMPROVED OXYGENATION AFTER OXYGEN ADMINISTRATION

Power of Added Oxygen

The great extent to which the arterial P_{O_2} can be increased by the inhalation of 100% oxygen is sometimes not appreciated. Suppose a young man has taken an overdose of an opiate drug that results in severe hypoventilation with an arterial P_{O_2} of 50 mm Hg and a P_{CO_2} of 80 mm Hg (see Figure 2.2). If this patient is mechanically ventilated and given 100% oxygen, the arterial P_{O_2} may increase to over 550 mm Hg, that is, a 10-fold increase (Figure 9.1). Few drugs can improve the gas composition of the blood so greatly and so effortlessly!

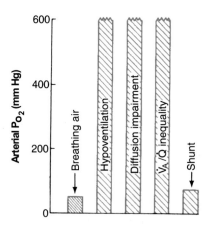

Figure 9.1. Response of the arterial P_{O_2} to 100% inspired oxygen for mechanisms of hypoxemia. The P_{O_2} breathing air is assumed to be 50 mm Hg. Note the dramatic increase in all instances except shunt where, nevertheless, there is a useful gain.

Response of Various Types of Hypoxemia

The mechanism of hypoxemia has an important bearing on the response to supplemental oxygen.

Hypoventilation

The rise in alveolar P_{O_2} can be predicted from the alveolar gas equation if the ventilation and metabolic rate, and therefore the alveolar P_{CO_2}, remain unaltered:

$$P_{A_{O_2}} = P_{I_{O_2}} - \frac{P_{A_{CO_2}}}{R} + F \qquad \text{(Eq. 9.1)}$$

where F is a small correction factor.

Assuming no change in the alveolar P_{CO_2} and the respiratory exchange ratio, and neglecting the correction factor, this equation shows that the alveolar P_{O_2} rises in parallel with the inspired value. Thus, changing from air to only 30% oxygen can increase the alveolar P_{O_2} by approximately 60 mm Hg. In practice, the arterial P_{O_2} is always lower than the alveolar value because of a small amount of venous admixture. However, the hypoxemia of hypoventilation, which is rarely severe, is easily reversed by a modest oxygen enrichment of the inspired gas. While oxygen is very effective in these cases, addressing the underlying cause of hypoventilation is an equally important intervention.

Diffusion Impairment

Hypoxemia caused by this mechanism is also readily overcome by oxygen administration. The reason for this becomes clear if we look at the dynamics of oxygen uptake along the pulmonary capillary (see Figure 2.4). The rate of movement of oxygen across the blood–gas barrier is proportional to the P_{O_2} difference between alveolar gas and capillary blood. (See *West's Respiratory Physiology: The Essentials*, 11th ed., p. 32.) This difference is normally approximately 60 mm Hg at the beginning of the capillary. If we increase the concentration of inspired oxygen to only 30%, we raise the alveolar P_{O_2} by 60 mm Hg, thus doubling the rate of transfer of oxygen at the start of the capillary. This in turn improves oxygenation of the end-capillary blood. Therefore, a modest rise in inspired oxygen concentration can usually correct the hypoxemia.

Ventilation–Perfusion Inequality

Oxygen administration usually is very effective at improving the arterial P_{O_2} in this situation too. However, the rise in P_{O_2} depends on the pattern of ventilation–perfusion inequality and the inspired oxygen concentration. Administration of an inspired oxygen fraction of 100% increases the arterial P_{O_2} to high values because every lung unit that is ventilated eventually washes out its nitrogen. When this occurs, the alveolar P_{O_2} is given by $P_{O_2} = P_B - P_{H_2O} - P_{CO_2}$. Because the P_{CO_2} is normally less than 50 mm Hg, this equation predicts an alveolar P_{O_2} of over 600 mm Hg, even in lung units with very low ventilation–perfusion ratios.

However, two cautions should be added. First, some regions of the lung may be so poorly ventilated that it may take several minutes for the nitrogen to be washed out. Furthermore, these regions may continue to receive nitrogen as this gas is gradually washed out of peripheral tissues by the venous blood. As a consequence, the arterial P_{O_2} may take so long to reach its final level that, in practice, this is never achieved. Second, giving oxygen may result in the development of unventilated areas (Figure 9.5), which limits the rise in the arterial P_{O_2} (Figure 9.3).

When intermediate concentrations of oxygen are given, the rise in arterial P_{O_2} is determined by the pattern of ventilation–perfusion inequality and in particular by those units that have low ventilation–perfusion ratios and appreciable blood flow. Figure 9.2 shows the response of the arterial P_{O_2} in lung models with various distributions of ventilation–perfusion ratios after inspiration of various oxygen concentrations. Note that at an inspired oxygen concentration of 60%, the arterial P_{O_2} of the distribution with a standard deviation of 2.0 rose from 40 to only 90 mm Hg. This modest rise can be attributed to the effects of lung units with ventilation–perfusion ratios less than 0.01. For example, an alveolus with a ventilation–perfusion ratio of 0.006 that is given 60% O_2

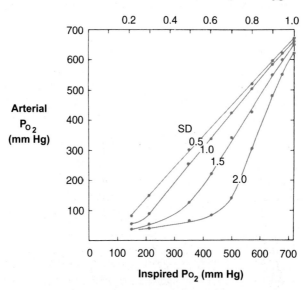

Figure 9.2. Response of the arterial P_{O_2} to various inspired oxygen values in theoretical distributions of ventilation–perfusion ratios. *SD* refers to the standard deviation of the log normal distribution. Note that when the distribution is broad (SD = 2), the arterial P_{O_2} remains low even when 60% oxygen is inhaled. (Republished with permission of Springer, from West JB, Wagner PD. Pulmonary gas exchange. In: West JB. ed. *Bioengineering Aspects of the Lung.* New York, NY: Marcel Dekker; 1977; permission conveyed through Copyright Clearance Center, Inc.)

to inspire has an end-capillary P_{O_2} of only 60 mm Hg in the example shown. However, note that when the inspired oxygen concentration was increased to 90%, the arterial P_{O_2} of this distribution rose to nearly 500 mm Hg.

Figure 9.2 assumes that the pattern of ventilation–perfusion inequality remains constant as the inspired oxygen is raised. However, the relief of alveolar hypoxia in poorly ventilated regions of the lung may increase the blood flow there because of the abolition of hypoxic pulmonary vasoconstriction. In this case, the increase in arterial P_{O_2} will be less. Note also that if units with low ventilation–perfusion ratios collapse during high oxygen breathing (Figure 9.5), the arterial P_{O_2} rises less.

Shunt

This is the only mechanism of hypoxemia in which the arterial P_{O_2} remains far below the level for the normal lung during 100% O_2 breathing. The reason is that the blood that bypasses the ventilated alveoli (shunt) does not "see" the added oxygen and, being low in oxygen concentration, depresses the arterial P_{O_2}. This depression is particularly marked because of the nearly flat slope of the oxygen dissociation curve at a high P_{O_2} (see Figure 2.6).

However, it should be emphasized that useful gains in arterial P_{O_2} often follow the administration of 100% O_2 to patients with shunts. This is because of the additional dissolved oxygen, which can be appreciable at a high alveolar P_{O_2}. For example, increasing the alveolar P_{O_2} from 100 to 600 mm Hg raises the dissolved oxygen in the end-capillary blood from 0.3 to 1.8 mL of O_2/100 mL of blood. This increase of 1.5 can be compared with the normal arterial–venous difference in oxygen concentration of approximately 5 mL/100 mL.

When hypoxemia is caused by shunt, the change in arterial P_{O_2} following increases in the inspired oxygen concentration varies based on the percentage shunt or shunt fraction (Figure 9.3). The graph is drawn for an oxygen uptake of 300 mL/min and a cardiac output of 6 L/min; variations in these and other

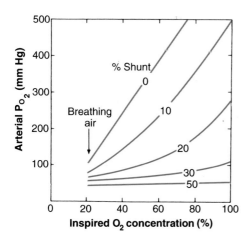

Figure 9-3. Response of the arterial P_{O_2} to increased inspired oxygen concentrations in a lung with various amounts of shunt. Note that the P_{O_2} remains far below the normal level for 100% oxygen. Nevertheless, useful gains in oxygenation occur even with severe degrees of shunting. (This diagram shows typical values only; changes in cardiac output, oxygen uptake, etc., affect the position of the lines.)

values alter the positions of the lines. In this example, if a patient with a 20% shunt and an arterial P_{O_2} of 55 mm Hg breathing air is given 100% oxygen, the arterial P_{O_2} will increase to 275 mm Hg. If, however, the patient had a 30% shunt, the P_{O_2} would only rise to 110 mm Hg with administration of the same inspired oxygen fraction. Depending on the clinical situation, however, even this smaller increase can raise the oxygen concentration enough to assist oxygen delivery.

Other Factors in Oxygen Delivery

Although the arterial P_{O_2} is a convenient measurement of the degree of oxygenation of the blood, other factors are important in oxygen delivery to the tissues. These factors include the hemoglobin concentration, the position of the oxygen dissociation curve, the cardiac output, and the distribution of the blood flow throughout the peripheral tissues.

Both a fall in hemoglobin concentration and cardiac output reduce the amount of oxygen per unit time ("oxygen flux") going to the tissues. The flux may be expressed as the product of the cardiac output and the arterial oxygen concentration: $\dot{Q} \times Ca_{O_2}$.

Diffusion of oxygen from the peripheral capillaries to the mitochondria in the tissue cells depends on capillary P_{O_2}. A useful index is the P_{O_2} of mixed venous blood, which reflects the average tissue P_{O_2}. A rearrangement of the Fick equation is as follows:

$$C\bar{v}_{O_2} = Ca_{O_2} - \frac{\dot{V}_{O_2}}{\dot{Q}} \qquad \text{(Eq. 9.2)}$$

This equation shows that the oxygen concentration (and therefore the P_{O_2}) of mixed venous blood will fall if either the arterial oxygen concentration or the cardiac output is reduced (oxygen consumption is assumed constant).

The relationship between oxygen concentration and P_{O_2} in the mixed venous blood depends on the position of the oxygen dissociation curve (see Figure 2.1). If the curve is shifted to the right by an increase in temperature, as in fever, or an increase in 2,3-diphosphoglycerate (DPG) concentration, as may occur in chronic hypoxemia, the P_{O_2} for a given concentration is high, thus favoring diffusion of oxygen to the mitochondria. By contrast, if the P_{CO_2} is low and the pH is high, as in respiratory alkalosis, or if the 2,3-DPG concentration is low because of transfusion of large amounts of stored blood, the resulting left-shifted curve interferes with oxygen unloading to the tissues.

Finally, the distribution of cardiac output clearly plays an important role in tissue oxygenation. For example, a patient who has coronary artery disease is liable to have hypoxic regions in the myocardium, irrespective of the other factors involved in oxygen delivery.

Important Factors in Oxygen Delivery to Tissues

- Arterial P_{O_2}
- Hemoglobin concentration
- Cardiac output
- Diffusion from capillaries to mitochondria (e.g., number of open capillaries)
- Oxygen affinity of hemoglobin
- Local blood flow

METHODS OF OXYGEN ADMINISTRATION

Oxygen can be administered by a variety of means. The appropriate method varies from patient to patient based on the clinical setting (e.g., at home versus in the hospital) and the severity of illness.

Nasal Cannulas

Nasal cannulas consist of two prongs that are inserted just inside the anterior nares and supported on a light frame. Oxygen is supplied at rates of 1 to 6 L/min, resulting in inspired oxygen concentrations of approximately 25% to 35%. The higher the patient's inspiratory flow rate, the lower the resulting concentration. When higher flow rates are used, the gas is often humidified to prevent patient discomfort and crusting of secretions on the nasal mucosa.

The chief advantage of cannulas is that the patient does not have the discomfort of a mask and he or she can talk and eat and has access to the face. The cannulas can be worn continuously for long periods, an important point because many patients with severe lung disease receive oxygen by nasal cannula on a chronic basis. The disadvantages of cannulas are the low maximum inspired concentrations of oxygen that are available and the unpredictability of the concentration, especially if the patient breathes with a high inspiratory flow rate or mostly through the mouth. This unpredictability can be minimized using a high-flow oxygen delivery system (see below).

Masks

Masks come in several designs. Simple plastic masks that fit over the nose and mouth allow inspired oxygen concentrations of up to 60% when supplied with flow rates of 10 to 15 L/min. Some patients report feeling smothered when this type of mask is used. Large holes in the side of the mask allow CO_2 to escape so it does not contribute to CO_2 retention.

Venturi masks are designed to deliver specific oxygen concentrations based on the Venturi effect. As oxygen enters the mask through a narrow jet, it entrains a constant flow of air, which enters via surrounding holes whose diameter can be adjusted to achieve the desired oxygen concentration. The smaller the diameter of the holes, the less ambient air in the gas mixture and the higher the inspired oxygen concentration. Masks that theoretically deliver inspired oxygen concentrations between 24% and 50% are available, but the true inspired concentration varies significantly between patients due to air leaks around the mask and variations in inspiratory flow rates.

Nonrebreather masks are designed to deliver high inspired oxygen concentrations approaching 80% to 100%. Oxygen is delivered at a flow rate of 10 to 15 L/min to a reservoir bag that hangs below the mask. Upon inhalation, the patient draws oxygen-enriched air from this reservoir into his or her respiratory tract. Exhaled air escapes via one-way valves in the side of the mask designed to prevent inhalation of ambient air and reinhalation of exhaled air. As with the simple and Venturi masks, air leaks and variations in inspiratory flow rate affect the delivered inspired oxygen concentration.

High-Flow Delivery Systems

Systems are now available for in-hospital use that deliver oxygen at very high flow rates through either a facemask or nasal cannula. By delivering gas at flow rates as high as 60 L/min, the systems limit the entrainment of ambient air that leads to unpredictability of inspired oxygen concentrations in the systems described above. High-flow nasal cannula systems are also thought to have the added benefit of improving ventilatory efficiency by flushing of the dead space in the upper airway and generating some positive end-expiratory pressure (PEEP). In well-selected patients with acute hypoxemic respiratory failure, use of these systems may obviate the need for invasive mechanical ventilation.

Transtracheal Oxygen

Oxygen can be delivered via a microcatheter inserted through the anterior tracheal wall with the tip lying just above the carina. Although it is an efficient way of delivering oxygen, particularly for patients on long-term oxygen therapy, its clinical use has fallen off significantly due improvements in ambulatory oxygen systems used in the care of patients with chronic lung disease.

Tents

These are now used for children who do not tolerate masks well. Oxygen concentrations of up to 50% can be obtained, but there is a fire hazard.

Ventilators

When a patient is mechanically ventilated through an endotracheal or tracheotomy tube, complete control over the composition of the inspired gas is available. There is a theoretical risk of producing oxygen toxicity if high inspired oxygen concentrations are given for more than a few days (see later). In general, the lowest inspired oxygen that provides an acceptable arterial P_{O_2} should be used. This level is difficult to define, but for most patients receiving invasive mechanical ventilation, a figure of 60 mm Hg is the typical goal. Increased levels of PEEP can also be applied to improve oxygenation in patients receiving invasive mechanical ventilation. This topic is discussed further in Chapter 10.

Extracorporeal Membrane Oxygenation

In patients with very severe respiratory failure, shunt and ventilation–perfusion inequality can be so severe that adequate oxygenation cannot be achieved despite use of mechanical ventilation with high inspired oxygen concentrations and PEEP. One approach in these situations is to oxygenate the blood outside the patient by placing them on extracorporeal membrane oxygenation (ECMO). In veno-venous (VV) ECMO, blood is removed through a cannula placed in a large vein (usually the femoral vein), passed through a membrane oxygenator with the aid of a centrifugal pump and then returned to the patient via a cannula in another large vein (usually the superior vena cava). In addition to oxygenating the blood, VV-ECMO facilitates removal of CO_2 and changes in ventilator settings that allow the injured lung to rest and recover.

Hyperbaric Oxygen

If 100% O_2 is administered at a pressure of 3 atmospheres, the inspired P_{O_2} is over 2,000 mm Hg. Under these conditions, a substantial increase in the arterial oxygen concentration can occur, chiefly as a result of additional dissolved oxygen. For example, if the arterial P_{O_2} is 2,000 mm Hg, the oxygen in solution is approximately 6 mL/100 mL of blood. Theoretically, this is enough to provide the entire arterial–venous difference of 5 mL/100 mL, so that the hemoglobin of the mixed venous blood could remain fully saturated.

Hyperbaric oxygen therapy has limited uses and is rarely indicated in the treatment of respiratory failure. However, it has been used in the treatment of severe carbon monoxide poisoning where most of the hemoglobin is unavailable to carry oxygen and therefore the dissolved oxygen is critically important. In addition, the high P_{O_2} accelerates the dissociation of carbon monoxide from hemoglobin. Severe anemic crises in patients who refuse blood transfusions are sometimes treated in the same way. Hyperbaric oxygen is also used in the treatment of severe decompression sickness, gas gangrene, nonhealing skin ulcers, as well as an adjunct to radiotherapy where the higher tissue P_{O_2} increases the radiosensitivity of relatively avascular tumors.

The use of hyperbaric oxygen requires a special facility with trained personnel. In practice, the chamber is filled with air, and oxygen is given by a special mask to ensure that the patient receives pure oxygen. This procedure also reduces fire hazard. Care is taken to avoid excessively high arterial P_{O_2}, which can provoke seizures.

Domiciliary and Portable Oxygen

Some patients are so disabled by severe chronic pulmonary disease that they have difficulty with any physical activity unless they breathe supplemental oxygen. These patients often benefit considerably from having a supply of oxygen in their home. Oxygen can be delivered using a large tank or an oxygen concentrator, which extracts oxygen from the air using a molecular sieve. Most patients also use portable oxygen sets to facilitate travel outside the home that use either liquid oxygen as a store or an oxygen concentrator.

The patients who benefit most from portable oxygen are those whose exercise tolerance is limited by dyspnea. Increasing the inspired oxygen concentration can greatly increase the level of exercise for a given ventilation and so enable these patients to become much more active.

It has been shown that a low flow of oxygen given continuously can reduce the amount of pulmonary hypertension and improve the prognosis of some patients with advanced chronic obstructive pulmonary disease (COPD). Although such therapy is expensive, improvements in the technology of providing oxygen have made it increasingly feasible for many patients.

MONITORING THE RESPONSE TO OXYGEN ADMINISTRATION

The response to oxygen administration can be assessed by looking for changes in a patient's clinical status such as improvements in mental status, cyanosis, the work of breathing, and dyspnea. A more precise method is to obtain an arterial blood gas that provides a direct assessment of the P_{O_2} and oxygen saturation, as well as information about ventilation and acid–base status. Because arterial blood can be difficult to obtain on a frequent basis, except for patients in an intensive care unit, the most common method of monitoring for hypoxemia and assessing the response to supplemental oxygen is pulse oximetry.

Oximeters operate based on the principle that hemoglobin transmits light differently depending on its degree of oxygenation. Two wavelengths of light are projected through the skin of either the finger or the ear lobe to a detector that measures the intensity of the transmitted light at each wavelength. The device then uses an internal algorithm to convert the signal to an estimate of the arterial oxygen saturation. Strong pulsatile blood flow is necessary for accurate measurements, as this allows the oximeter to distinguish light transmitted by hemoglobin in arterial blood from that transmitted by venous blood and other tissue elements. The accuracy of an oximeter is not as good as co-oximetry performed on an arterial blood gas, but its convenience makes it valuable in the clinical setting.

HAZARDS OF OXYGEN THERAPY

Carbon Dioxide Retention

The reasons for the development of dangerous CO_2 retention after excessive oxygen administration to patients with severe COPD or the obesity hypoventilation syndrome were briefly discussed in Chapter 8. A critical factor in the ventilatory drive of these patients who have a high work of breathing is often the hypoxic stimulation of their peripheral chemoreceptors. If this is removed by relieving their hypoxemia, the level of ventilation may fall precipitously and severe CO_2 retention may ensue. Relief of hypoxic pulmonary vasoconstriction and changes in ventilation–perfusion matching also play an important role.

In patients with CO_2 retention, intermittent use or abrupt cessation of supplemental oxygen can lead to severe hypoxemia. The explanation is that if oxygen administration is seen to cause CO_2 retention and is abruptly stopped, the subsequent hypoxemia may be more severe than it was before oxygen therapy. The reason is the increased alveolar P_{CO_2}, as can be seen from the alveolar gas equation:

$$P_{A_{O_2}} = P_{I_{O_2}} - \frac{P_{A_{CO_2}}}{R} + F \qquad \text{(Eq. 9.3)}$$

This shows that any increase in alveolar P_{CO_2} will reduce the alveolar P_{O_2} and therefore the arterial value. Moreover, the high P_{CO_2} is likely to remain for many minutes because the body stores of this gas are so great that the excess is washed out only gradually. Thus, the hypoxemia may be severe and prolonged.

To avoid this problem, patients with chronic CO_2 retention should be given continuous oxygen at a low-enough concentration to achieve an oxygen saturation of 88% to 94%, with monitoring of ventilation using end-tidal CO_2 monitoring or arterial blood gases. The shape of the oxygen dissociation curve (see Figure 2.1) should be at the back of the physician's mind to remind him or her that a rise in P_{O_2} from 30 to 50 mm Hg (at a normal pH) represents more than a 25% increase in hemoglobin saturation!

Oxygen Toxicity

Animal studies have demonstrated that high concentrations of oxygen over long periods damage the lung. Studies of monkeys exposed to 100% oxygen for 2 days show that some of the earliest changes are in the capillary endothelial cells, which become swollen. Alterations occur in the endothelial intercellular junctions, and there is an increased capillary permeability that leads to interstitial and alveolar edema. In addition, the alveolar epithelium may become denuded and replaced by rows of type 2 epithelial cells. Later, organization occurs with interstitial fibrosis.

The extent to which these changes occur in humans is difficult to determine, but normal subjects report substernal discomfort after breathing 100% oxygen for 24 hours. Patients who have been mechanically ventilated with 100% oxygen for 36 hours have shown a progressive fall in arterial P_{O_2} compared with a control group who were ventilated with air. Recent clinical studies have also suggested that clinical outcomes are worsened for patients whose arterial P_{O_2} is maintained at too high a level for excessive periods of time.

The risks of using high inspired oxygen concentrations with high-flow nasal cannula or mechanical ventilation must be balanced against the need to maintain adequate arterial oxygenation in patients with severe hypoxemic respiratory failure. For this reason, the general practice is to use the lowest inspired oxygen concentration necessary to maintain an adequate arterial P_{O_2}.

Atelectasis

Following Airway Occlusion

If a patient is breathing air and an airway becomes totally obstructed, for example, by retained secretions, absorption atelectasis of the lung behind the airway may occur. The reason is that the sum of the partial pressures in the venous blood is considerably less than atmospheric pressure, with the result that the trapped gas is gradually absorbed. (See *West's Respiratory Physiology: The Essentials*, 11th ed., pp. 180-181.) However, the process is relatively slow, requiring many hours or even days.

However, if the patient is breathing a high concentration of oxygen, the rate of absorption atelectasis is greatly accelerated. This is because there is then relatively little nitrogen in the alveoli and this gas normally slows the absorption process because of its low solubility. Replacing the nitrogen with any other gas that is rapidly absorbed also predisposes to collapse. An example is nitrous oxide during anesthesia. In the normal lung, collateral ventilation may delay or prevent atelectasis by providing an alternative path for gas to enter the obstructed region (see Figure l.11C).

Absorption atelectasis is common in patients with respiratory failure because they often have excessive secretions or cellular debris in their airways and they are frequently treated with high oxygen concentrations. In addition, the channels through which collateral ventilation normally occurs may be obstructed by disease. Collapse is common in the dependent regions of the lung because secretions tend to collect there, and those airways and alveoli are relatively poorly expanded anyway (see Figure 3.3). Hypoxemia develops to the extent that atelectatic lung is perfused, although hypoxic pulmonary vasoconstriction may limit this to some extent.

Instability of Units with Low Ventilation–Perfusion Ratios

It has been shown that lung units with low ventilation–perfusion ratios may become unstable and collapse when high oxygen mixtures are inhaled. An example is given in Figure 9.4, which shows the distribution of ventilation–perfusion ratios in a patient during air breathing and after 30 minutes of 100% oxygen. This patient had respiratory failure after a motor vehicle collision (see Figure 8.4). Note that during air breathing there were appreciable

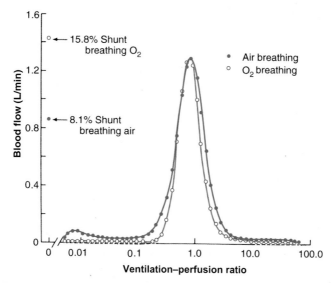

Figure 9.4. **Conversion of low ventilation–perfusion ratio units to shunt during oxygen breathing.** This patient had respiratory failure after motor vehicle collision. During air breathing, there was appreciable blood flow to units with low ventilation–perfusion ratios. After 30 minutes of 100% oxygen, blood flow to these units was not evident, but the shunt doubled.

amounts of blood flow to lung units with low ventilation–perfusion ratios in addition to an 8% shunt. After oxygen administration, the blood flow to the low ventilation–perfusion ratio units was not evident, but the shunt had increased to nearly 16%. The most likely explanation for this change is that the poorly ventilated regions became unventilated.

Figure 9.5 shows the mechanism involved. The figure shows four hypothetical lung units, all with low inspired ventilation–perfusion ratios ($\dot{V}_A/\dot{Q}$) during 80% oxygen breathing. In A, the inspired (alveolar) ventilation is 49.4 units but the expired ventilation is only 2.5 units (the actual values depend on the blood flow). The reason why so little gas is exhaled is that so much is taken up by the blood. In B, where the inspired ventilation is slightly reduced to 44.0 units (same blood flow as before), there is no expired ventilation because all the gas that is inspired is absorbed by the blood. Such a unit is said to have a "critical" ventilation–perfusion ratio.

In Figure 9.5C and D, the inspired ventilation has been further reduced with the result that it is now less than the volume of gas entering the blood. This is an unstable situation. Under these circumstances, either gas is inspired from neighboring units during the expiratory phase of respiration, as in C, or the unit gradually collapses, as in D. The latter fate is particularly likely if the unit is poorly ventilated because of intermittent airway closure. This is probably common in the dependent regions of the lung in ARDS because of the greatly reduced FRC. The likelihood of atelectasis increases rapidly as the inspired oxygen concentration approaches 100%.

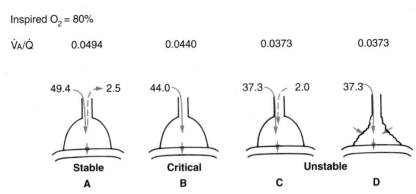

Inspired $O_2 = 80\%$

$\dot{V}_A/\dot{Q}$ 0.0494   0.0440   0.0373   0.0373

49.4 → 2.5   44.0   37.3 — 2.0   37.3

Stable   Critical   Unstable

A   B   C   D

Figure 9.5. **Mechanism of the collapse of lung units with low inspired ventilation–perfusion ratios ($\dot{V}_A/\dot{Q}$) when high oxygen mixtures are inhaled. A.** The expired ventilation is very small because so much of the inspired gas is taken up by the blood. **B.** There is no expired ventilation because all of the ventilation is taken up by the blood. **C,D.** More gas is removed from the lung unit than is inspired, leading to an unstable condition.

The development of shunts during oxygen breathing is an additional reason to avoid, if possible, high concentrations of this gas in the treatment of patients with respiratory failure. Also, the shunt that is measured during 100% oxygen breathing (see Figure 2.6) in these patients may substantially overestimate the shunt that is present during air breathing.

Retinopathy of Prematurity

If premature infants with the infant respiratory distress syndrome are treated with high concentrations of oxygen, they may develop fibrosis behind the lens of the eye, leading to retinal detachment and blindness. Formerly known as retrolental fibroplasia, this problem can be prevented by avoiding overly high arterial P_{O_2} and other established risk factors.

KEY CONCEPTS

1. Oxygen therapy is extremely valuable in the treatment of many patients with lung disease, and it can often greatly increase the arterial P_{O_2}.

2. The response of the arterial P_{O_2} to inhaled oxygen varies considerably depending on the cause of the hypoxemia. Patients with large shunts do not respond well, although even here a small increase in arterial P_{O_2} can be helpful.

3. Various methods of oxygen administration are available. Nasal cannulas are valuable for long-term treatment of patients with COPD. The highest inspired oxygen concentrations are obtained with intubation and mechanical ventilation.

4. Hazards of oxygen therapy include oxygen toxicity, carbon dioxide retention, atelectasis, and retinopathy of prematurity.

CLINICAL VIGNETTE

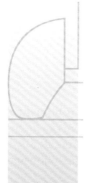

A 41-year-old man presents with 2 days of fevers, productive cough, and worsening dyspnea. On examination, he is febrile, laboring to breathe, and has an S_pO_2 of 80% breathing ambient air. He has dullness to percussion and decreased breath sounds in the left lower lung zone. A chest radiograph shows a large, dense opacity involving the entire left lower lobe. On his laboratory studies, his WBC is 15×10^3 cells/µL (normal 4 to 10×10^3 cells/µL) and hemoglobin 7 g/dL (normal 13 to 15 g/dL). An arterial blood gas at the time of presentation shows a P_{CO_2} of 34 mm Hg and P_{O_2} of 55 mm Hg. After his oxygen saturation fails to improve on oxygen by nasal cannula and then a nonrebreather mask, he is intubated and placed on mechanical ventilation with an F_IO_2 of 1.0. An arterial blood gas performed following intubation demonstrates a P_{O_2} of 62 mm Hg.

Questions

- How do you explain the observed change in his P_{O_2} following initiation of mechanical ventilation?
- What effect will his fever have on tissue oxygen delivery?
- What change would you expect to see in the oxygen content of the mixed venous blood compared to his normal healthy state?
- What interventions besides mechanical ventilation with a high inspired oxygen concentration can be considered to improve tissue oxygen delivery?

QUESTIONS

For each question, choose the one best answer.

1. A previously healthy woman is brought to the Emergency Department following an opiate overdose that caused severe hypoventilation. If she receives supplemental oxygen with an F_IO_2 of 0.5 and there is no change in her arterial P_{CO_2}, by how much would you expect her arterial P_{O_2} (in mm Hg) to increase?
   A. 25
   B. 50
   C. 75
   D. 100
   E. 200

2. A patient with congenital heart disease and a right-to-left shunt of 20% of the cardiac output has an arterial P_{O_2} of 60 mm Hg while breathing

ambient air. If you were to administer supplemental oxygen with an F_IO_2 of 1.0, which of the following responses would you expect to see in the arterial P_{O_2}?

A. Decrease by 10 mm Hg
B. Increase by less than 10 mm Hg
C. Increase by more than 10 mm Hg
D. Increase to 570 mm Hg
E. No change

3. After being pulled out of a burning house, a 32-year-old man is brought into the Emergency Department where co-oximetry performed on an arterial blood gas sample while he was breathing ambient air reveals a carboxyhemoglobin level of 25% (normal: <1%). Which of the following would you expect to see as a result of this finding?

A. Decreased P_{50} for hemoglobin
B. Decrease red blood cell 2,3-DPG concentration
C. Increased arterial pH
D. Increased arterial oxygen content
E. Increased mixed venous P_{O_2}

4. A patient with normal lungs but severe anemia is placed in a hyperbaric chamber, total pressure 3 atmospheres, and 100% oxygen is administered by valve box. You can expect the dissolved oxygen in the arterial blood (in mL O_2 per 100 mL blood) to increase to:

A. 2
B. 4
C. 6
D. 10
E. 15

5. A 77-year-old man with very severe COPD is admitted to the hospital with an exacerbation of his disease. After he is placed on 6 L/min of oxygen by nasal cannula, his S_pO_2 increases from 80% breathing air to 99%. Two hours later, he is noted to be more somnolent and an arterial blood gas reveals that his arterial P_{CO_2} rose from 48 mm Hg on admission to 79 mm Hg. Which of the following statements best explains the observed change in his arterial P_{CO_2}?

A. Decreased peripheral chemoreceptor stimulation of ventilation
B. Improved ventilation–perfusion matching
C. Increased arterial pH
D. Increased formation of carbamino groups on the hemoglobin chains
E. Rightward shift of the hemoglobin–oxygen dissociation curve

6. The distribution of ventilation–perfusion ratios for a patient with respiratory failure is shown in the figure below. The panel on the left displays the ratios when the patient is breathing ambient air, while the

panel on the right displays the ratios after 90 minutes breathing gas with an inspired oxygen fraction (F_IO_2) of 1.0.

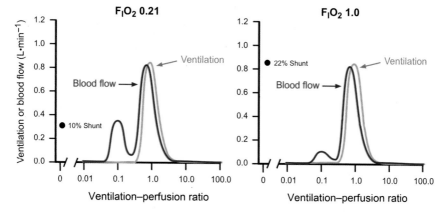

Which of the following best accounts for the observed change in the distribution of ventilation–perfusion ratios after breathing air with an F_IO_2 of 1.0?

A. Alveolar edema due to oxygen toxicity
B. Faster removal of alveolar gas by blood than replacement by ventilation
C. Inactivation of surfactant
D. Small airway closure due to accumulation of interstitial edema
E. Small airway inflammation and smooth muscle contraction

7. A patient presents to the Emergency Department and requires intubation and initiation of invasive mechanical ventilation for severe acute respiratory failure. Arterial blood gases obtained before and after intubation are shown in the table below.

Timing	F_IO_2	Arterial P_{CO_2} (mm Hg)	Arterial P_{O_2} (mm Hg)
Preintubation	0.21	32	62
Postintubation	1.0	34	100

Based on these data, which of the following is the most likely cause of hypoxemia in this patient?

A. Diffusion impairment
B. Hypoventilation
C. Shunt
D. Ventilation–perfusion inequality

8. A right heart catheter is placed on a 70-year-old woman admitted to the intensive care unit with pulmonary edema following an exacerbation of heart failure with reduced ejection fraction. She is receiving supplemental oxygen by high-flow nasal cannula. The cardiac output, arterial P_{O_2}, and hemoglobin concentration are measured before (Time 1) and after (Time 2) administration of the inotrope dobutamine. The results are shown in the table below.

Time	Cardiac output (L/min)	Arterial P_{O_2} (mm Hg)	Hemoglobin (g/dL)
1	2.4	62	12.1
2	3.6	69	12.0

Which of the following would you expect to see at Time 2 compared to Time 1?
A. Decreased rate of diffusion of oxygen from the capillaries to the mitochondria
B. Decreased plasma pH
C. Decreased tissue oxygen consumption ($\dot{V}O_2$)
D. Increased mixed venous oxygen concentration
E. Lactic acidosis

9. A 52-year-old woman presents to the Emergency Department with 2 days of productive cough, fever, and worsening dyspnea. On evaluation, her oxygen saturation is 80% breathing ambient air, and she is using accessory muscles of respiration, appears to have a high inspiratory flow rate, and has decreased breath sounds and dullness to percussion at her right lung base. Which of the following oxygen delivery systems is most likely to deliver the intended inspired oxygen fraction in this situation?
A. High-flow nasal cannula
B. Nonrebreather mask
C. Simple face mask
D. Standard nasal cannula
E. Venturi mask

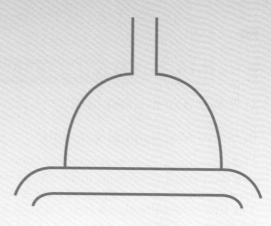

Mechanical Ventilation

10

Mechanical ventilation is frequently employed to improve oxygenation and ventilation in patients with various causes of respiratory failure. It is a complex and technical subject, and this discussion is limited to the physiologic principles of its use, benefits, and hazards. At the end of this chapter, the reader should be able to:

- Describe the operating principles of the basic modes of mechanical ventilation
- Describe the benefits and risks of increased positive end-expiratory pressure (PEEP)
- Predict the effects of changes in ventilator settings on the dead space fraction
- Describe the effects of mechanical ventilation on the pulmonary capillaries, venous return, and oxygen delivery
- List the hazards of mechanical ventilation

METHODS OF MECHANICAL VENTILATION

Mechanical ventilation can be delivered to patients through a variety of means.

Invasive Mechanical Ventilation

Many patients with acute respiratory failure are supported through invasive mechanical ventilation in which the ventilator is connected to the upper airway via an endotracheal or, less commonly, a tracheotomy tube. The latter is usually placed after a patient has been endotracheally intubated for a long period of time but is occasionally placed at the onset of respiratory failure when the upper airway is compromised by, for example, anaphylaxis or a laryngeal tumor. Endotracheal tubes can be inserted via the nose or mouth. Endotracheal and tracheotomy tubes include an inflatable cuff at the distal end to give an airtight seal. With either type of tube, the lungs are inflated by delivering positive pressure to the airway (Figure 10.1).

Noninvasive Mechanical Ventilation

Positive pressure can also be applied to the airway using a tight-fitting mask around the patient's nose and mouth. This noninvasive form of support is

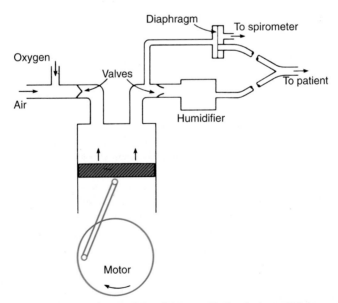

Figure 10.1. Example of a constant volume ventilation (schematic). In practice, the tidal volume and frequency can be regulated. During the expiratory phase, as the piston descends, the diaphragm is deflected to the left by the reduced pressure in the cylinder, allowing the patient to exhale through the spirometer.

increasingly being used in critical care, particularly for patients with ventilatory failure due to the obesity hypoventilation syndrome or acute exacerbations of chronic obstructive pulmonary disease. In fact, for the latter, it is preferred over invasive mechanical ventilation as the initial means for supporting ventilation in patients with severely impaired mechanics. It is not an effective form of support, however, for patients with severe hypoxemic respiratory failure due to pneumonia or ARDS and is generally avoided in patients who cannot protect their airway, who have excessive respiratory secretions or who are at high risk for aspiration.

Tank Ventilators

Unlike with the methods described above, tank respirators deliver negative pressure (less than atmospheric) to the outside of the chest and rest of the body, excluding the head. They consist of a rigid box (iron lung) connected to a large-volume, low-pressure pump that controls the respiratory cycle. The box is often hinged along the middle so that it can be opened to allow nursing care.

Tank ventilators are no longer used in the treatment of acute respiratory failure because they limit access to the patient and because they are bulky and inconvenient. They were employed extensively to ventilate patients with bulbar poliomyelitis, and they are still occasionally useful for patients with chronic neuromuscular disease who need to be ventilated for months or years. A modification of the tank ventilator is the cuirass, which fits over the thorax and abdomen and also generates negative pressure. It is usually reserved for patients who have partially recovered from neuromuscular respiratory failure.

WHEN TO INITIATE MECHANICAL VENTILATION

The decision to initiate mechanical ventilation should not be lightly undertaken because it is a major intervention that requires a substantial investment of personnel and equipment, with many hazards. There are no specific numerical thresholds for the arterial P_{CO_2} or P_{O_2} that mandate mechanical support. Instead, the timing of mechanical ventilation is dictated by a variety of factors, including the severity of the disease process, the rapidity of the progress of hypoxemia and hypercapnia, and the hemodynamic stability and general condition of the patient.

MODES OF MECHANICAL VENTILATION

The majority of modern ventilators can deliver positive-pressure ventilation by a variety of means, referred to as "modes" of ventilation. The appropriate mode for a given patient varies based on their clinical and physiologic needs.

The most commonly used modes are described below. More detailed information about these and other modes of mechanical ventilation can be found in textbooks on critical care medicine.

Volume Control

A preset volume is delivered to the patient at a specified rate. However, patients who are not receiving neuromuscular blockading medications or who are not too heavily sedated and have normal respiratory muscles can initiate breaths beyond the set rate and receive the full tidal volume with each extra breath. The ratio of inspiratory to expiratory time can be adjusted by changing the inspiratory flow rate. This can be particularly useful in patients with obstructive lung disease for whom it is important to ensure adequate time for exhalation. The pressure required to deliver a breath is determined by the chosen flow rate and tidal volume, the airway resistance and compliance, and the positive end-expiratory pressure (PEEP, described further below).

This mode has the advantage of having a known volume delivered to the patient despite changes in the elastic properties of the lung or chest wall or increases in airway resistance. A disadvantage is that delivery of the intended volume may require high distending pressures, which can be injurious to the lung. However, in practice, a safety blow-off valve prevents pressure from reaching dangerous levels.

Pressure Control

Rather than delivering a constant tidal volume with each breath, this mode delivers a preset pressure for a specified duration of time. A minimum frequency is set, but patients can initiate breaths beyond the specified rate, during which they receive the preset pressure. The flow of gas is not set by the practitioner and, instead, is determined by the change in pressure on inhalation and airway resistance. The ratio of inspiratory to expiratory time is controlled by adjusting the inspiratory time.

The advantage of this mode is that it prevents development of excessive airway pressure. The chief disadvantage is that the volume of gas delivered with each breath can vary with changes in the compliance of the respiratory system. Also, an increase in airway resistance may decrease the ventilation because there may be insufficient time for equilibration of pressure between the machine and the alveoli. Minute ventilation must therefore be monitored closely.

Pressure Support

This mode is similar to pressure control in that the patient receives a preset pressure during inhalation. However, there is no preset rate, and the patient must initiate all of the breaths. As such, it is only suitable for patients who are able to initiate breathing. In addition, rather than being turned off after a preset time, the inspiratory pressure is terminated once inspiratory flow falls below a certain threshold. This mode, which is commonly used for patients who require intubation solely to prevent aspiration of oral or gastric secretions or are having difficulty being liberated from the ventilator due to neuromuscular weakness, is generally more comfortable for patients.

A variant of this mode, referred to as bi-level positive airway pressure, is commonly used during noninvasive mechanical ventilation. When the patient initiates a breath, the inspiratory pressure is raised to and maintained at a preset level, referred to as the inspiratory positive airway pressure (IPAP) until inspiratory flow decreases. During exhalation, airway pressure is maintained at a level above zero cm H_2O, referred to as the expiratory positive airway pressure (EPAP), which serves the same function as PEEP.

Continuous Positive Airway Pressure

In this mode, a constant positive pressure is applied to the airway by the ventilator during inhalation and exhalation. This improves oxygenation by increasing FRC and preventing atelectasis. Continuous positive airway pressure (CPAP) is commonly used in patients being weaned from ventilator breathing or who are intubated solely for airway protection.

It can also be applied to patients through a tight fitting mask or nasal interfaces, as is done in neonates with neonatal respiratory distress syndrome (see Chapter 8) or adults with pulmonary edema due to a heart failure exacerbation.

High-Frequency Ventilation

In high-frequency jet or oscillatory ventilation, very low tidal volumes (50 to 100 mL) are delivered at a high frequency (approximately 20 cycles per second). The lung is vibrated rather than expanded in the conventional way, and the transport of the gas occurs by a combination of diffusion and convection. Because it maintains higher mean airway pressures than more conventional ventilator modes, high-frequency ventilation is sometimes used in patients with severe ARDS, although this practice is more common in children than adults. Another use is in patients with gas leaks from the lung via a bronchopleural fistula.

POSITIVE END-EXPIRATORY PRESSURE

For most patients receiving mechanical ventilation, 5 cm H_2O of pressure is applied to the airways during exhalation. This is referred to as positive end-expiratory pressure (PEEP) and is intended to counteract the decrease in functional residual capacity and atelectasis that can occur when patients are ventilated in the supine or semirecumbent position. Rather than being a mode of mechanical ventilation per se, it is an intervention that can be used in most modes of mechanical ventilatory support.

When the arterial P_{O_2} does not rise despite increased inspired oxygen concentrations, as can happen in patients with large shunts due to severe pneumonia or ARDS (see Figure 9.3), PEEP is often raised to levels higher than 5 cm H_2O as a means to improve gas exchange. In some cases, pressures as high as 20 cm H_2O may be used. PEEP tends to be most effective for improving oxygenation in diffuse bilateral processes, such as ARDS or pulmonary edema, and less effective with focal processes such as pneumonia involving a single lobe or segment of the lung.

Several mechanisms are probably responsible for the increase in arterial P_{O_2} with increased PEEP. The positive pressure increases the transmural pressure and, as a result, increases FRC, which is typically small in these patients because of the increased elastic recoil of the lung (Figure 10.2). By doing so, PEEP reverses the low lung volumes that lead to airway closure, intermittent or absent ventilation, and absorption atelectasis, especially in the dependent regions (see Figures 3.3 and 9.5). Patients with edema in their airways also benefit, probably because the fluid is moved into small peripheral airways or alveoli, allowing some regions of the lung to be reventilated. A secondary gain from PEEP is that by increasing the arterial P_{O_2}, it may allow the inspired oxygen concentration to be decreased, thus lessening the risk of oxygen toxicity.

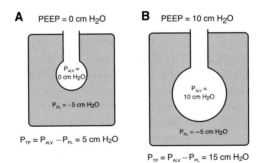

Figure 10.2. The effect of PEEP on transpulmonary pressure and alveolar volume. With application of PEEP, alveolar pressure (P_{ALV}) increases. This increases the difference between the alveolar and pleural (P_{PL}), referred to as the transpulmonary pressure (P_{TP}). For a given compliance, this increases alveolar volume. Note that the pleural pressure is assumed to remain constant for the purposes of simplicity, but in practice, it may increase following the application of PEEP.

> ### Positive End-Expiratory Pressure (PEEP)
>
> - Increases FRC and prevents atelectasis
> - 5 cm H_2O used in most patients receiving mechanical ventilation
> - Higher levels useful for raising the arterial P_{O_2} in patients with respiratory failure
> - Values up to and above 20 cm H_2O can be used in cases of severe hypoxemia
> - May allow the inspired O_2 concentration to be reduced

PHYSIOLOGIC EFFECTS OF MECHANICAL VENTILATION

Reduction of Arterial P_{CO_2}

A major role of mechanical ventilation is to assist ventilation and decrease the P_{CO_2} in patients who are not able to breathe spontaneously, as in neuromuscular disease or a drug overdose, or who have severely diseased lungs, as in ARDS. In patients with airway obstruction in whom the oxygen cost of breathing is high, mechanical ventilation may appreciably reduce the oxygen uptake and CO_2 output, thus contributing to the fall in arterial P_{CO_2}.

The relationship between the arterial P_{CO_2} and the alveolar ventilation in normal lungs is given by the alveolar ventilation equation:

$$P_{CO_2} = \frac{\dot{V}_{CO_2}}{\dot{V}_A} \cdot K \qquad \text{(Eq. 10.1)}$$

where K is a constant. In diseased lungs, the denominator $\dot{V}_A$ in this equation is less than the ventilation going to the alveoli because of alveolar dead space, that is, unperfused alveoli or those with high ventilation–perfusion ratios. For this reason, the denominator is sometimes referred to as the "effective alveolar ventilation."

Mechanical ventilation frequently increases both the alveolar and anatomic dead spaces. As a consequence, the effective alveolar ventilation is not increased as much as the total ventilation. This is particularly likely if high pressures are applied to the airway. This can be seen in the example shown in Figure 10.3. As the level of PEEP was increased from 0 to 16 cm H_2O in this patient with ARDS, the dead space increased from 36.3% to 49.8%. In some patients, high levels of PEEP also result in the appearance of lung units with high ventilation–perfusion ratios that cause a shoulder to form on the right of the ventilation distribution curve. This did not occur in the example shown. Occasionally, a large physiologic dead space is seen with positive-pressure ventilation even in the absence of PEEP.

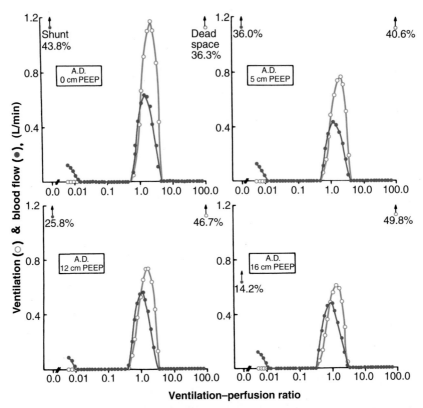

Figure 10.3. Reduction of shunt and increase of dead space caused by increasing levels of PEEP in a patient with adult respiratory distress syndrome (ARDS). Note that as the PEEP was progressively increased from 0 to 16 cm H_2O, the shunt decreased from 43.8% to 14.2% of the cardiac output, and the dead space increased from 36.3% to 49.8% of the tidal volume. (Rerpinted from Dantzker DR, Brook CJ, DeHart P, et al. Ventilation–perfusion distributions in the adult respiratory distress syndrome. *Am Rev Respir Dis.* 1979;120(5):1039–1052. Copyright © 1979 American Thoracic Society. All Rights Reserved.)

There are several reasons why positive-pressure ventilation increases dead space. First, lung volume is usually raised, especially when PEEP is added, and the resulting radial traction on the airways increases the volume of anatomic dead space. Next, the raised airway pressure tends to divert blood flow away from ventilated regions, thus causing areas of high ventilation–perfusion ratio or even unperfused areas (Figure 10.4). This is particularly likely to happen in the uppermost regions of the lung where the pulmonary artery pressure is relatively low because of the hydrostatic effect. (See *West's Respiratory Physiology: The Essentials*, 11th ed., p. 54.) Indeed, if the pressure in the capillaries falls below airway pressure, the capillaries may collapse completely, resulting in unperfused lung (Figure 10.4). This collapse is encouraged by two factors: (1) the abnormally high airway pressure and (2) the reduced venous return

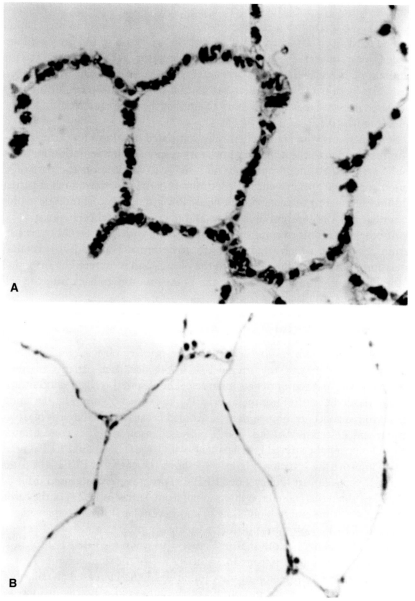

Figure 10.4. Effect of raised airway pressure on the histologic appearance of pulmonary capillaries. A. Normal appearance. **B.** Collapse of capillaries when alveolar pressure is raised above capillary pressure. (Reprinted from Glazier JB, Hughes JMB, Maloney JE, et al. Measurements of capillary dimensions and blood volume in rapidly frozen lungs. *J Appl Physiol*. 1969;26(1):65–76. Copyright © 1969 by American Physiological Society. All rights reserved.)

and consequent hypoperfusion of the lung. The latter is particularly likely to occur if there is a reduced circulating blood volume (see later in this chapter).

The tendency for the arterial P_{CO_2} to rise as a result of the increased dead space can be countered by increasing the respiratory rate to increase the total ventilation. Nevertheless, it is important to remember that an increase in mean airway pressure can cause a substantial rise in dead space, although the increased pressure may be necessary to combat the shunt and resulting hypoxemia (Figure 10.3).

Some patients who are mechanically ventilated develop a low arterial P_{CO_2}. This may be due to the hypoxic ventilatory response, compensation for a metabolic acidosis, an inappropriately high drive to breathe on the part of the patient, or inappropriate ventilator settings. In some situations, such as patients with intracranial hypertension, an unduly low arterial P_{CO_2} should be avoided because it reduces cerebral blood flow and may cause cerebral hypoxia.

Another hazard of overventilation of patients with CO_2 retention is a low serum potassium, which predisposes to arrhythmia. When CO_2 is retained, potassium moves out of the cells into the plasma and is excreted by the kidney. If the P_{CO_2} is then rapidly reduced, the potassium moves back into the cells, thus depleting the plasma.

Increase in Arterial P_{O_2}

In many patients with respiratory failure, the primary objective of mechanical ventilation is to increase the arterial P_{O_2}. In practice, such patients are always ventilated with oxygen-enriched mixtures. The inspired oxygen concentration should ideally be set to raise the arterial P_{O_2} to at least 60 mm Hg, but unduly high inspired concentrations should be avoided because of the hazards of oxygen toxicity and atelectasis. As noted above, increased inspired oxygen concentrations may not increase the arterial P_{O_2} in patients with large shunts, and PEEP is necessary to improve the situation. Figure 10.3 shows the effects of PEEP in a patient with ARDS. Note that the level of PEEP was progressively increased from 0 to 16 cm H_2O, and this caused the shunt to fall from 43.8% to 14.2% of the cardiac output. A small amount of blood flow to poorly ventilated alveoli remained.

While PEEP is often useful for reducing shunt, it can also lead to unintended consequences. Note that in Figure 10.3, increased PEEP also caused the dead space to increase from 36.3% to 49.8% of the tidal volume. This can be explained by compression of the capillaries by the increased alveolar pressure and also the increase in volume of the lung and consequent increased radial traction on the airways, which increases their volume.

Occasionally, the addition of too much PEEP reduces rather than increases the arterial P_{O_2}. One important mechanism is a substantial fall in cardiac output on high levels of PEEP, which reduces the P_{O_2} of mixed venous blood and therefore the arterial P_{O_2}. PEEP tends to reduce cardiac output by impeding venous return to the thorax, especially if the circulating blood volume has been depleted by hemorrhage or shock. Accordingly, the effect of PEEP should not be gauged by the change in the arterial P_{O_2} alone but in terms of the total amount of oxygen delivered to the tissues. The product of the arterial oxygen concentration and the cardiac output is a useful index because changes in this alter the P_{O_2} of mixed venous blood and therefore the P_{O_2} of many tissues. An alternative approach to assess the adequacy of oxygen delivery is to draw blood from a central venous catheter and measure the central venous oxygen saturation, a surrogate measure of the mixed venous value.

Other mechanisms by which PEEP may reduce the P_{O_2} include reduced ventilation of well-perfused regions (because of increasing dead space and ventilation to poorly perfused regions) and diversion of blood flow away from ventilated to unventilated regions by the raised airway pressure. The latter problem is often observed when PEEP is used in processes with focal, rather than diffuse, lung involvement.

Another hazard of high levels of PEEP is damage to the pulmonary capillaries as a result of the high tension in the alveolar walls. The alveolar wall can be considered a string of capillaries. High levels of tension greatly increase the stresses on the capillary walls, causing disruption of the alveolar epithelium, capillary endothelium, or sometimes all layers of the wall. This is another example of "stress failure," which was discussed in Chapter 6 in relation to pulmonary edema caused by high capillary hydrostatic pressures.

Effects on Venous Return

As noted above, mechanical ventilation tends to impede the return of blood into the thorax and thus reduce the cardiac output and systemic blood pressure. In patients with severe pulmonary hypertension, where maintenance of adequate preload is critical for preserving right ventricular function, the decrease in venous return with initiation of mechanical ventilation can have severe hemodynamic consequences, such as systemic hypotension.

The effect of mechanical ventilation on venous return is true for both positive-pressure and negative-pressure ventilation. In a supine, relaxed patient, the return of blood to the thorax depends on the difference between the peripheral venous pressure and the mean intrathoracic pressure. If the airway pressure is increased by the ventilator, mean intrathoracic pressure rises, thereby decreasing the pressure gradient for venous return. Even if airway pressure remains atmospheric, as in a tank respirator, venous return tends to fall because the peripheral venous pressure is reduced by the negative pressure. Only with the cuirass respirator is venous return virtually unaffected.

The effects of positive-pressure ventilation on venous return depend on several factors. The most important of these are the magnitude and duration of the inspiratory pressure, particularly on the addition of PEEP. The ideal pattern from this standpoint is a short inspiratory phase of relatively low pressure followed by a long expiratory phase and ideally zero (or slightly negative) end-expiratory pressure. However, such a pattern leads to low lung volume and, as a result, hypoxemia, and a compromise is generally necessary.

The 5 cm H_2O of PEEP given to most patients receiving mechanical ventilation generally has little effect on venous return.

Another important determinant of venous return is the magnitude of the circulating blood volume. If this is reduced, for example, by hemorrhage or hyopvolemic shock, positive-pressure ventilation often causes a marked fall in cardiac output, leading to systemic hypotension. It is therefore important to correct any volume depletion by appropriate fluid replacement. Ultrasound and central venous pressure monitoring can be used to guide such fluid administration. The latter should be interpreted in the light of the increased airway pressure, as positive airway pressure itself raises central venous pressure.

Venous return may also decrease due to a process referred to as "auto-PEEP." If the patient is unable to completely exhale the delivered tidal volume with each breath, progressive hyperinflation can develop leading to an increase in intrathoracic pressure and decreased venous return. This process can be seen in patients intubated during COPD or asthma exacerbations or patients ventilated with very high respiratory rates (e.g., as compensation for a severe metabolic acidosis), which are associated with decreased exhalation time.

Miscellaneous Hazards

A variety of other problems can be seen with mechanical ventilation. *Mechanical problems* are a constant hazard. They include power failure, microprocessor malfunctions, broken connections, and kinking of tubes. Mechanical ventilators are equipped with a variety of alarms to warn of these dangers, but skilled care by the intensive care team is essential.

Barotrauma can occur, especially if high levels of PEEP and/or unusually large tidal volumes are used. Air that ruptures out of the alveolar space can enter the pleural space, causing *pneumothorax*, or track along the perivascular and peribronchial interstitium (see Figure 6.1), and enter the mediastinum (*pneumomediastinum*). Air that enters the mediastinum can track further along tissue planes to the subcutaneous tissue of the neck and chest wall (*subcutaneous emphysema*).

Excessive tidal volumes can also cause *ventilator-induced lung injury* due to repetitive overstretching of the alveoli. Careful attention to ensure patients do not receive tidal volumes more than 8 mL/kg of the body weight predicted based on their sex and height is critical for preventing this problem.

Ventilator-associated pneumonia can develop in patients who remain on mechanical ventilation for more than a short period. *Cardiac arrhythmias* may be caused by rapid swings in pH and hypoxemia. There is also an increased incidence of *gastrointestinal bleeding* in these patients who are not receiving enteral nutrition while being ventilated.

Several complications are associated with endotracheal and tracheotomy tubes. Ulceration of the larynx or the trachea is sometimes seen, particularly if the inflated cuff exerts undue pressure on the mucosa. This can lead to scarring and tracheal stenosis, damage to the cartilaginous rings in the trachea and development of a tracheoesophageal fistula. The use of large-volume, low-pressure cuffs has reduced the incidence of these problems considerably.

Care must be taken with the placement of an endotracheal tube to avoid inadvertent placement of the distal end of the tube in the right main bronchus (*right mainstem intubation*), which can cause atelectasis of the left lung and often the right upper lobe.

KEY CONCEPTS

1. Mechanical ventilation has a major role in treating patients with respiratory failure. Ventilatory support can be delivered invasively through endotracheal tube or a tracheotomy tube or noninvasively through a tight-fitting mask.

2. Most ventilators support patients through positive-pressure ventilation. Negative-pressure, or tank, ventilators are now seldom used except for patients with long-term neuromuscular disease.

3. There are multiple modes for delivering positive-pressure ventilation. These modes are frequently combined with positive end-expiratory pressure (PEEP) to improve oxygenation in patients with severe hypoxemia.

4. Mechanical ventilation, especially when used with an increased oxygen concentration and PEEP, typically increases the arterial P_{O_2} and reduces the P_{CO_2}. However, it can reduce venous return and may cause barotrauma and other complications.

CLINICAL VIGNETTE

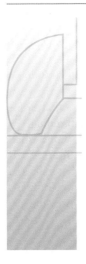

A 54-year-old woman presents to the Emergency Department with 2 days of dyspnea, fever, productive cough, and pleuritic right-sided chest pain. After a chest radiograph demonstrates a right lower lobe opacity, she is diagnosed with pneumonia and admitted to the hospital ward. Although she was started on appropriate antibiotic therapy, she develops increased difficulty with her breathing and hypoxemia and requires transfer to the ICU. Despite use of high flow oxygen in the ICU, she remains hypoxemic and requires intubation and initiation of invasive mechanical ventilation. A chest radiograph done following intubation now shows diffuse bilateral opacities. She is started on volume control ventilation with a tidal volume of 550 mL, a respiratory rate of 20, F_IO_2 1.0, and PEEP 5 cm H_2O. The following data were obtained before and 30 minutes following intubation:

(Continued)

CLINICAL VIGNETTE (*Continued*)

Time Point	Blood Pressure (mm Hg)	Arterial P_{O_2} (mm Hg)	Arterial P_{CO_2} (mm Hg)
Preintubation	130/77	51	46
Postintubation	98/69	58	38

Questions
- How do you account for the observed change in her arterial P_{CO_2} following intubation?
- What changes would you expect to occur in her dead space following intubation?
- What effect will the findings on chest radiography have on the pressure needed to inflate her lungs on inhalation?
- What intervention can you consider to improve her oxygenation?
- How do you account for the decrease in her blood pressure following intubation?

QUESTIONS

For each question, choose the one best answer.

1. A 40-year-old man is receiving invasive mechanical ventilation for severe ARDS. He is ventilated using the volume control mode with a rate of 15 breath per minute, tidal volume of 500 mL, and PEEP 5 cm H_2O. After increasing the F_IO_2 from 0.5 to 1.0, his arterial P_{O_2} remained less than 60 mm Hg. Which of the following interventions is most appropriate to improve his oxygenation?
   A. Change to pressure control ventilation
   B. Increase the inspiratory flow rate
   C. Increase the PEEP
   D. Increase the respiratory rate
   E. Increase the tidal volume

2. A 66-year-old woman is intubated to prevent aspiration of blood after presenting with hemorrhagic shock due to upper gastrointestinal bleeding. She is placed on volume control ventilation with an F_IO_2 of 0.5 and tidal volume of 450 mL. Following intubation, her blood pressure falls from 110/70 to 85/50 mm Hg. On examination, she has equal breath sounds bilaterally and her trachea remains in the midline position. Which of the following is most likely responsible for the observed change in her blood pressure?
   A. Decreased venous return
   B. Hypercarbia
   C. Placement of the endotracheal tube into the right mainstem bronchus
   D. Pneumothorax
   E. Resorption atelectasis

3. You are looking at the ventilator being used on a patient intubated for severe respiratory failure. The machine is set to deliver 10 breaths per minute, but the patient is receiving a total of 18 breaths per minute. With each breath, the pressure is increased 10 cm H_2O above the set PEEP and maintained at that level for 1 second. The volume delivered appears to vary over time. Which of the following modes is being used to ventilate the patient?
   A. Continuous positive airway pressure
   B. High-frequency oscillatory ventilation
   C. Pressure control
   D. Pressure support
   E. Volume control

4. A patient with paralyzed respiratory muscles but normal lungs is receiving invasive mechanical ventilation. Which of the following interventions can be used to reduce the arterial P_{CO_2} without changing total ventilation?
   A. Increase the inspired oxygen fraction
   B. Increase the respiratory frequency
   C. Increase the tidal volume
   D. Reduce the functional residual capacity
   E. Reduce the airway resistance

5. A patient is receiving invasive mechanical ventilation for management of severe community-acquired pneumonia complicated by the acute respiratory distress syndrome. In response to worsening oxygenation, the PEEP was increased from 12 to 18 cm H_2O. The distribution of ventilation–perfusion ratios on each level of PEEP are displayed in the figure below.

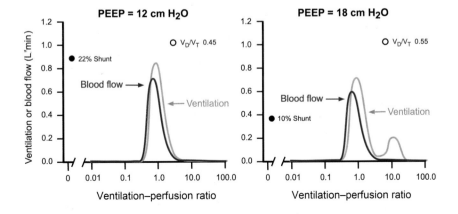

Which of the following most likely accounts for the observed changes on a PEEP of 18 cm H_2O?
A. Compression of alveolar capillaries
B. Decreased pulmonary vascular resistance
C. Decreased radial traction on the airways
D. Increased airway resistance
E. Increased venous return

6. A 71-year-old man with a long history of tobacco use presents to the Emergency Department with increasing dyspnea. Pulmonary function tests performed several weeks earlier in clinic revealed an FEV_1 55% predicted, FVC 65% predicted, and FEV_1/FVC of 0.57. On examination in the emergency department, he has an S_pO_2 of 80% breathing air, is using accessory muscles of respiration, and has diffuse expiratory wheezes and a prolonged expiratory phase on lung auscultation. A chest radiograph shows large lung volumes, flattened diaphragms but no focal opacities while an arterial blood gas demonstrates a pH of 7.21, a P_{CO_2} of 61 mm Hg, and a P_{O_2} of 52 mm Hg. Which of the following is the most appropriate initial intervention for this patient at this time?
A. High flow nasal cannula
B. Invasive mechanical ventilation
C. Noninvasive positive-pressure ventilation
D. Nonrebreather mask
E. Venturi mask

7. After presenting with traumatic brain injury following a fall off a ladder, a patient is intubated and started on invasive mechanical ventilation to prevent aspiration of oral secretions. He is placed on volume control ventilation with a tidal volume of 8 mL/kg, a respiratory rate of 10 breaths per minute, inspired oxygen fraction of 1.0, and a PEEP of 5 cm H_2O. A chest radiograph performed shortly after intubation reveals atelectasis of the left lung and the right upper lobe. Which of the following is most likely responsible for the findings on chest radiography?
A. Decreased venous return
B. Resorption atelectasis
C. Respiratory alkalosis
D. Right mainstem intubation
E. Ventilator-induced lung injury

8. A patient is receiving invasive mechanical ventilation after presenting with a myocardial infarction. A pulmonary artery catheter was inserted following admission to monitor cardiac output. In response to worsening oxygenation, the PEEP was increased from 10 to 15 cm H_2O.

The arterial P$_{O_2}$, hemoglobin concentration, and mixed venous oxygen content before and after this intervention are shown in the table below.

PEEP (cm H$_2$O)	Arterial P$_{O_2}$ (mm Hg)	Hemoglobin (g/dL)	Mixed Venous Oxygen Content (mL O$_2$/100 mL)
10	50	13.3	14
15	55	13.4	12

Which of the following best accounts for the observed changes in the mixed venous oxygen content?
A. Decreased cardiac output
B. Decreased pulmonary vascular resistance
C. Increased airway resistance
D. Increased venous return
E. Pneumomediastinum

SYMBOLS, UNITS, AND NORMAL VALUES

SYMBOLS

Primary

C   Concentration of gas in blood
F   Fractional concentration in dry gas
P   Pressure or partial pressure
Q   Volume of blood
$\dot{Q}$ Volume of blood per unit time
R   Respiratory exchange ratio
S   Saturation of hemoglobin with O_2
V   Volume of gas
$\dot{V}$ Volume of gas per unit time

Secondary Symbols for Gas Phase

A   Alveolar
B   Barometric
D   Dead space
E   Expired
I   Inspired
L   Lung
T   Tidal

Secondary Symbols for Blood Phase

a   Arterial
c   Capillary
c'   End-capillary
i   Ideal
v   Venous
$\bar{v}$ Mixed venous

Examples

O_2 concentration in arterial blood: Ca_{O_2}
Fractional concentration of N_2 in expired gas: $F_{E_{N_2}}$
Partial pressure of O_2 in mixed venous blood: $P\overline{v}_{O_2}$

UNITS

Traditional metric units are used in this book. Pressures are given in mm Hg; the torr is an almost identical unit.

In Europe, SI (Système International) units are now commonly used. Most of them are familiar, but the kilopascal, the unit of pressure, is confusing at first. One kilopascal = 7.5 mm Hg (approximately).

Conversion of Gas Volumes to BTPS

Lung volumes, including FEV_1 and FVC, are conventionally expressed at body temperature (37°C), ambient pressure, and saturated with water vapor (BTPS). To convert volumes measured in a spirometer at ambient temperature (t), pressure, saturated (ATPS) to BTPS,

$$\frac{310}{273+t} \cdot \frac{P_B - P_{H_2O}(t)}{P_B - 47}$$

In practice, tables are available for this conversion.

The derivation of this equation and all the other equations is given in the companion volume (see *West's Respiratory Physiology: The Essentials*, 11th ed., p. 214).

REFERENCE VALUES

Reference Values for Lung Function Tests

Normal values depend on age, sex, height, weight, and ethnicity. This is a complex subject; for a detailed discussion, see pages 333–365 of Cotes JE, Chinn DJ, Miller MR. *Lung Function*. 6th ed. Oxford, UK: Blackwell; 2006. Representative reference values for some common tests are shown in Table A.1. Pulmonary function laboratories may use different reference values based on other data sets and, as a result, predicted values may vary from those shown in this table.

Table A.1   Example of Reference Values for Common Pulmonary Function Tests in Nonsmoking Adults in the United States

	Men	Women
TLC (L)	7.95 St^a + 0.003 A^b − 7.33 (0.79)^c	5.90 St − 4.54 (0.54)
FVC (L)	7.74 St − 0.021 A − 7.75 (0.51)	4.14 St − 0.023 A − 2.20 (0.44)
RV (L)	2.16 St + 0.021 A − 2.84 (0.37)	1.97 St + 0.020 A − 2.42 (0.38)
FRC (L)	4.72 St + 0.009 A − 5.29 (0.72)	3.60 St + 0.003 A − 3.18 (0.52)
RV/TLC (%)	0.309 A + 14.1 (4.38)	0.416 A + 14.35 (5.46)
FEV_1 (L)	5.66 St − 0.023 A − 4.91 (0.41)	2.68 St − 0.025 A − 0.38 (0.33)
FEV_1/FVC (%)	110.2 − 13.1 St − 0.15 A (5.58)	124.4 − 21.4 St − 0.15 A (6.75)
$FEF_{25\%-75\%}$ (L/s)	5.79 St − 0.036 A − 4.52 (1.08)	3.00 St − 0.031 A − 0.41 (0.85)
$MEF_{50\% \, FVC}$ (L/s)	6.84 St − 0.037 A − 5.54 (1.29)	3.21 St − 0.024 A − 0.44 (0.98)
$MEF_{25\% \, FVC}$ (L/s)	3.10 St − 0.023 A − 2.48 (0.69)	1.74 St − 0.025 A − 0.18 (0.66)
DI (mL/min/ mm Hg)	16.4 St − 0.229 A + 12.9 (4.84)	16.0 St − 0.111 A + 2.24 (3.95)
DI/V_A	10.09 − 2.24 St − 0.031 A (0.73)	8.33 − 1.81 St − 0.016 A (0.80)

[a]St is stature (height) (m).
[b]A is age (years).
[c]Standard deviation is in parentheses.

FURTHER READING

Broaddus VC, Mason RJ, Ernst JD, King TE, Lazarus SC, Murray JF, Nadel JA, Slutsky AS, Gotway MB. *Murray and Nadel's Textbook of Respiratory Medicine*. 7th ed. Philadelphia, PA: Elsevier; 2020.

Crystal RG, West JB, Weibel ER, Barnes PJ. *The Lung: Scientific Foundations*. 2nd ed. Philadelphia, PA: Lippincott-Raven; 1997.

Grippi MA, Elias JA, Fishman JA, Kotloff RM, Pack AI, Senior RM. *Fishman's Pulmonary Diseases and Disorders*. 5th ed. New York, NY: McGraw-Hill Education; 2015.

Kumar V, Abbas AK, Aster JC. *Robbins and Cotran Pathologic Basis of Disease*. 10th ed. Philadelphia, PA: W.B. Saunders Co.; 2021.

ANSWERS TO END-OF-CHAPTER QUESTIONS

CHAPTER 1

Question 1. A is correct. Compared to the healthy individual, the patient has a reduced FEV_1 and a reduced FVC. In addition, a large portion of the total exhaled volume came out in the first second. This pattern is consistent with restrictive disease. Of the diseases on the list, the one that could cause this pattern would be pulmonary fibrosis, a disease marked by scarring of the lung tissue. Asthma, chronic bronchitis, and emphysema would demonstrate an obstructive pattern in which the FEV_1 is reduced and represents a small percentage of the total exhaled volume (i.e., a low FEV_1/FVC ratio). Chronic thromboembolic pulmonary hypertension, a pulmonary vascular disease, does not cause changes on spirometry.

Question 2. C is correct. The presence of a reduced FEV_1 and FVC with a decreased FEV_1/FVC ratio indicates that this patient has airflow obstruction. Given the long history of smoking and the findings on examination and chest radiography, this is most likely related to chronic obstructive pulmonary disease, which in turn could be due to emphysema and/or chronic bronchitis. These patients are prone to premature collapse of the airways on exhalation, particularly forced exhalation, due to loss of elastic recoil and decreased radial traction on the airways. This results in airway closure at a higher lung volume and, therefore, a higher closing volume. The expiratory limb of the flow volume loop often has a scooped out appearance (Figure 1.5B) and would not be flatted in COPD. Peak expiratory flow and the $FEF_{25\%-75\%}$ are typically reduced. These patients often have uneven ventilation, and, as a result, the slope of phase 3 of the single-breath nitrogen washout is increased.

Question 3. C is correct. The single-breath nitrogen washout provides information about whether a patient has uneven ventilation. The phase 3 slope—often referred to as the alveolar plateau—is nearly flat in healthy individuals, whereas it is increased in those with uneven ventilation. Of the items on the list, the one that could cause this is increased airway secretions, as these increase resistance and delay emptying of the affected regions. The arterial partial pressures of oxygen and carbon dioxide and the hemoglobin concentration do not contribute to regional differences in ventilation throughout the lung. Airway walls may be thickened in chronic bronchitis. While emphysema may lead to enlargement of air spaces, it does not cause thinning of the airway walls.

Question 4. B is correct. This woman has airflow obstruction on spirometry as evidenced by the low FEV_1/FVC ratio. This develops due to dynamic compression of the airways. Lung compliance is increased in emphysema, while radial traction on the airways is decreased due to the loss of elastic recoil, and the blood–gas barrier has normal thickness. The diaphragm is not weak in these patients, although contractile efficiency may be diminished due to hyperinflation.

Question 5. D is correct. Although smokers commonly develop obstructive lung disease, the spirometry is consistent with a restrictive process, such as pulmonary fibrosis. Asthma, chronic bronchitis, and chronic obstructive pulmonary disease would cause airflow obstruction, while pulmonary hypertension is typically associated with normal spirometry.

Question 6. E is correct. Better effort on spirometry leads to increased peak expiratory flow but will not change flow at end-exhalation when flow is limited by dynamic airway compression. Vital capacity would be expected to increase with better effort, while flattening of the expiratory and inspiratory limbs of the flow–volume loops occurs with various forms of upper airway obstruction rather than as a function of patient effort.

Question 7. D is correct. The flow–volume loop has a "scooped out" appearance often seen in patients with airflow obstruction. Of the items on the list of choices, increased airway secretions is the one that could cause airflow obstruction by increasing airway resistance. Fibrosis of the lung parenchyma and increased elastic recoil would be associated with normal flows but decreased vital capacity. Increased radial traction on the airways would improve rather than limit airflow, while the number of pulmonary capillaries has no effect on spirometry.

Question 8. B is correct. The chest radiograph shows severe kyphoscoliosis, a deformity of the spine marked by curvature in the coronal and sagittal planes. This problem causes restrictive ventilatory impairment. On pulmonary function testing, this would manifest with a reduced FVC and FEV_1, but the FEV_1/FVC ratio would be normal, as most of the expired volume comes out in the first second. Decreased $FEF_{25-75\%}$, decreased FEV_1/FVC, and increased closing volume are typically seen in obstructive diseases. The expiratory and inspiratory limbs of the flow–volume loop are flattened with fixed (i.e., nonvariable) upper airway obstruction.

CHAPTER 2

Question 1. D is correct. With administration of supplemental oxygen with an F_IO_2 of 1.0, the arterial P_{O_2} increased to only 300 mm Hg. In healthy individuals, the arterial P_{O_2} should increase to about 570 mm Hg when breathing this inspired oxygen fraction. Of the primary causes of hypoxemia, the only one in which the arterial P_{O_2} will not rise to the normal level seen in healthy individuals with an F_IO_2 of 1.0 is shunt. For all of the other causes, the Pa_{O_2} should normalize, although this may not be the case in some patients with chronic obstructive pulmonary disease because it can take nitrogen a long time to wash out of very poorly ventilated alveoli. The fact that the patient's father and brother had a similar problem suggests that he may have a genetic disorder. Confirming the presence of shunt raises concern he could have an arteriovenous malformation, a feature of a genetic disorder known as hereditary hemorrhagic telangiectasia (see Chapter 6).

Question 2. D is correct. The patient has hypoxemia and an increased alveolar–arterial oxygen difference (39 mm Hg). This is seen with ventilation–perfusion inequality. It can also be seen in shunt, but this was not an answer choice. Hypoventilation is not present given the normal arterial P_{CO_2}, while low P_IO_2 is ruled out because she is at sea level. Diffusion impairment does not cause hypoxemia in individuals at rest at sea level.

Question 3. E is correct. Because there was no change in the dead space volume, when the tidal volume was decreased from 750 to 450 mL, the alveolar volume decreased to from 600 to 300 mL. Given that the respiratory rate remained constant at 10 breaths per minute, the alveolar ventilation ($\dot{V}_A$) decreased from 6,000 to 3,000 mL/min. Looking at the alveolar ventilation equation (Equation 2.1), we see that the arterial P_{CO_2} is inversely proportional to $\dot{V}_A$. Because $\dot{V}_A$ fell by 50%, we can expect the P_{CO_2} to double, that is the new value will be 200% of its original value.

Question 4. D is correct. The history of excessive daytime somnolence and report of excessive snoring, grunts, and gasps while sleeping at night is highly suggestive of a diagnosis of obstructive sleep apnea, a common form of sleep-disordered breathing that causes intermittent hypoxemia. Untreated individuals are at risk for a variety of adverse cardiovascular outcomes including hypertension, coronary artery disease, and cerebrovascular disease that develop as a result of sympathetic nervous system activation in response to the apneic periods and endothelial dysfunction. None of the other problems listed among the answer choices are consequences of untreated sleep apnea.

Question 5. B is correct. The histopathologic image from the lung biopsy shows markedly thickened alveolar walls. This finding can be seen in patients with pulmonary fibrosis. This creates a barrier to diffusion, which, on pulmonary function testing, will manifest as a reduction in the diffusing capacity for carbon monoxide. Increased total lung capacity, increased closing volume, and decreased FEV_1/FVC ratio are all findings that might be seen in a patient with chronic obstructive pulmonary disease due to emphysema and/ or chronic bronchitis. The forced vital capacity would be decreased, rather than increased, in a patient with thickening of the alveolar walls like that seen in the image.

Question 6. D is correct. The patient's FEV_1/FVC ratio and TLC are normal, while the diffusion capacity for carbon monoxide is decreased. This can occur due to anemia as the decreased hemoglobin concentration leads to decreased uptake of carbon monoxide across the alveolar–capillary barrier during the test. Asthma and chronic obstructive pulmonary disease cause reductions in the FEV_1/FVC ratio, while idiopathic pulmonary fibrosis decreases TLC, and sarcoidosis has variable effects on pulmonary function testing.

Question 7. B is correct. The arterial blood gas demonstrates a primary metabolic acidosis with respiratory compensation, which can be seen in diabetic ketoacidosis. Chronic obstructive pulmonary disease exacerbation, morbid obesity, and opiate overdoses would be associated with primary respiratory acidoses, while severe vomiting would cause a primary metabolic alkalosis.

Question 8. B is correct. With ascent to high altitude, the pressure gradient for diffusion across the alveolar–capillary barrier is diminished. This will slow the rate of rise of the P_{O_2} in the pulmonary capillaries. Individuals hyperventilate following ascent due to increased peripheral chemoreceptor stimulation. This leads to a respiratory rather than a metabolic alkalosis. The shunt fraction does not change following ascent while the diffusion capacity for carbon monoxide might actually increase due to increased blood flow through the pulmonary capillaries due to the increase in cardiac output.

Question 9. A is correct. The figure demonstrates that the average alveolar P_{O_2} is higher than normal, while the average alveolar P_{CO_2} is lower than normal. This pattern is consistent with that seen in hyperventilation. Of the items on the list, the one associated with hyperventilation is an anxiety attack. Each of the choices are situations in which you might see hypoventilation. An opiate overdose leads to a suppression of respiratory drive, while COPD exacerbations are associated with worsening lung mechanics and subsequent inability to maintain adequate minute and alveolar ventilation. Guillain-Barré syndrome and poliomyelitis both cause neuromuscular weakness, which impairs the individual's ability to maintain sufficient minute and alveolar ventilation.

Question 10. D is correct. Progressive, ascending weakness following a diarrheal infection caused by *Campylobacter jejuni* raises concern for a diagnosis of Guillain-Barré syndrome, a form of ascending paralysis that can eventually involve the muscles of respiration. The fact that she has hypoxemia and her vital capacity is reduced suggests that she is now developing respiratory impairment. Respiratory muscle problems due to neuromuscular disease manifest as hypoventilation, the hallmark of which is an increase in the arterial P_{CO_2}. This would be associated with a decrease in pH and, depending on the duration of hypoventilation, an increase in her serum bicarbonate. The alveolar P_{O_2} is reduced with hypoventilation. The diffusion capacity for carbon monoxide should remain largely unchanged since the lung parenchyma itself is unaffected, although small decreases can sometimes be seen if atelectasis develops due to the hypoventilation.

CHAPTER 3

Question 1. E is correct. The slope of the relationship between volume and pressure is decreased in the patient compared to the healthy control. This indicates that lung compliance is reduced. Of the items on the list, the one that can do this is pulmonary fibrosis, a diffuse parenchymal lung disease marked by deposition of fibrotic tissue in the lung parenchyma. Asthma, chronic bronchitis, and emphysema would typically be associated with increased compliance, while pulmonary arterial hypertension should not affect compliance as it is largely a disease of the pulmonary vasculature rather than the lung parenchyma.

Question 2. E is correct. The ventilation–perfusion scan shows an area of lung that receives ventilation but no perfusion. This finding occurs in pulmonary embolism. Asthma and chronic obstructive pulmonary disease exacerbations would cause heterogeneity on the ventilation images but not the perfusion images, while pneumothorax might show impaired ventilation and perfusion in the same region. Myocardial infarction would not affect the ventilation or perfusion images.

Question 3. A is correct. The arrow denotes total lung capacity. Airway resistance is at its lowest value at this volume because the expansion of the lung parenchyma exerts traction on the airway walls. Transpulmonary pressure and elastic recoil are both at their maximum values at high lung volumes. Pulmonary vascular resistance is lowest at functional residual capacity and increases at the extremes of lung volume. Arterial pH would not be expected to change significantly in a single forced expiration maneuver.

Question 4. E is correct. Functional residual capacity is determined by the balance of the recoil of the lung and chest wall. In a patient with evidence of obstructive lung disease due to emphysema, the functional residual capacity would increase due to decreased lung recoil. Airway resistance, total lung capacity, and lung compliance are often increased in these individuals, while the diffusion capacity for carbon monoxide is decreased.

Question 5. B is correct. When healthy individuals perform a cardio-pulmonary exercise test, heart rate typically increases to greater than 80% of the maximum predicted value (220-age), R typically rises above 1.0 due to an increase in CO_2 elimination following onset of lactic acidosis, minute ventilation increases, and arterial P_{CO_2} decreases as part of respiratory compensation for a metabolic acidosis. The decrease in arterial P_{O_2} from 90 to 65 mm Hg would be considered an atypical response, as this parameter usually remains constant in healthy individuals over the course of progressive exercise.

Question 6. B is correct. Plethysmography measures all the gas in the lung, while the helium dilution technique "sees" only those regions of lung that communicate with the mouth. Therefore, regions behind closed airways result in a higher value for the plethysmographic than for the dilution procedure. This phenomenon can be seen in patients with chronic obstructive pulmonary disease but not the other diseases on the list.

Question 7. C is correct. This patient has a markedly increased body mass index (BMI) and a compensated respiratory acidosis on arterial blood gas, indicative of ongoing hypoventilation. This clinical picture is consistent with a diagnosis of the obesity hypoventilation syndrome. As with patients with chronic CO_2 retention due to severe COPD, these patients often have depressed ventilatory responses to CO_2. Even though the patient is hypoxemic, the ventilatory response to hypoxemia is typically not increased and, instead, is often decreased. Closing volume may be increased in very obese individuals due to early airway closure at the lung bases. Decreased residual volume is often seen in parenchymal lung disease that causes increased radial traction on the airways and would not be expected in an individual with no opacities on chest radiography. There is no history to support a diagnosis of emphysema or asthma that might lead to increased pulmonary compliance.

Question 8. B is correct. The distributions of ventilation and perfusion are affected by gravity. As one moves from the base to the apex of the lung, both ventilation and perfusion decrease. Because perfusion decreases to a greater extent than ventilation, the average ventilation–perfusion ratio increases as one moves toward the apex of the lung. High ventilation–perfusion units, and therefore, the apex of the lung, have increased alveolar P_{O_2} and decreased alveolar P_{CO_2} when compared to low ventilation–perfusion units at the base of the lungs.

Question 9. A is correct. There are several important findings in the results of the exercise test. The arterial P_{CO_2} increased over the course of the test, while the arterial P_{O_2} decreased. Also, the heart rate at maximum exercise is far below his predicted maximum, while the minute ventilation is quite close to the predicted maximum. R also does not rise above 1, and the lactate is only minimally increased, both of which suggest the individual did not reach his anaerobic (i.e., ventilatory) threshold. All of these findings, but most importantly, the rising P_{CO_2} over the course of exercise, suggest that the patient has problems with his ventilatory pump. Of the items on the list of answer choices, the one that could lead to this pattern of results is chronic obstructive pulmonary disease. These individuals often develop severe air trapping with exercise, which impairs ventilatory mechanics. They cannot ventilate enough to eliminate the CO_2 being produced with exercise and overcome their high physiologic dead space. Thus, P_{CO_2} rises over the course of the test. The fact that the minute ventilation is close to the predicted maximum also suggests the ventilatory pump reached the limits of its capacity.

CHAPTER 4

Question 1. E is correct. In young individuals, episodic dyspnea and chest tightness triggered by exercise is highly suggestive of a diagnosis of asthma. The increase in symptoms and frequency of inhaler use that prompted the clinic visit, as well as the diffuse wheezing on examination, indicate he is having an exacerbation. Air trapping is more extensive during exacerbations, and, as a result, one would expect to see increased residual volume (RV). All of the other parameters would decrease in patients whose asthma control is worsening.

Question 2. C is correct. The key finding in the CT scan of the chest is a marked enlargement in the airspaces of the lung. This is a common finding in emphysema, the primary cause of which is excess release of lysosomal elastase by neutrophils leading to destruction of elastin, a critical structural protein for the lung. Bronchial smooth muscle hypertrophy and hyperplasia and airway wall infiltration by eosinophils and lymphocytes are key features of asthma, which is not accompanied by lung parenchymal changes on chest imaging such as those seen in the figure. Excess collagen deposition in the interstitial space is seen in pulmonary fibrosis, while long-standing unresolved bronchial obstruction leads to bronchiectasis. Neither of these diseases demonstrate the appearance seen in the CT images in this patient.

Question 3. A is correct. The distribution of ventilation–perfusion ratios in Patient 1 indicates that there is a large amount of blood flow to low $\dot{V}_A/\dot{Q}$ units, whereas in Patient 2, there is little blood flow to such units and, instead, a large amount of ventilation to high $\dot{V}_A/\dot{Q}$ units. Because it is the low $\dot{V}_A/\dot{Q}$ units that causes hypoxemia rather than high $\dot{V}_A/\dot{Q}$ units, you would expect to see more hypoxemia with Patient 1. This demonstrates some of the variation in physiologic and clinical features that can be seen in individuals with COPD.

Question 4. C is correct. The information provided indicates this patient has chronic obstructive pulmonary disease. When caused by emphysema, this is associated with decreased vascular markings on chest radiography. The retrosternal airspace is typically enlarged in these patients. Bilateral hilar lymphadenopathy is associated with sarcoidosis and lymphoma, while reticular opacities are seen with diffuse pulmonary fibrosis and bilateral opacities are seen in pulmonary edema.

Question 5. C is correct. This young woman has asthma that is not under adequate control. Because asthma is an inflammatory disorder, she should begin daily use of an inhaled corticosteroid. Inhaled long-acting β_2-agonists should not be used as the primary controller medication unless a patient is already on inhaled steroids. The other medications listed would not be appropriate as the first-line controller medication.

Question 6. E is correct. This patient has airflow obstruction on pulmonary function testing, which can be seen with all of the answer choices. The findings on chest radiography suggest this patient has emphysema. Several features fit with this being due to panacinar emphysema (likely due to alpha-one antitrypsin deficiency) rather than centriacinar disease, including the fact that he developed it at a young age, has only a modest smoking history, and has extrapulmonary involvement (small, nodular liver). Centriacinar emphysema due to cigarette smoking tends to primarily affect the upper lobes and presents at a later age. Asthma is unlikely given the lack of a bronchodilator response and the findings on chest radiography. Chronic bronchitis is unlikely given the lack of productive cough, while an obstructing lesion in the trachea is unlikely based on the lack of stridor and findings on the chest radiograph.

Question 7. E is correct. This woman has chronic obstructive pulmonary disease. Air trapping commonly leads to an increased residual volume in these patients and an increased RV/TLC ratio. Functional residual capacity is increased due to decreased lung recoil, while diffusion capacity for carbon monoxide is decreased due to the loss of surface area for gas exchange. The total lung capacity is often increased due to air trapping and hyperinflation.

Question 8. E is correct. Ventilation–perfusion inequality is the predominant cause of hypoxemia in patients with acute severe asthma. Shunt can occur when there is mucous plugging of the airways, and this may contribute to her hypoxemia. She is not hypoventilating at this time. Hyperventilation would actually increase the arterial P_{O_2} in the absence of ventilation–perfusion inequality. Diffusion impairment is not a cause of hypoxemia in these patients.

Question 9. B is correct. The numerical data from the pulmonary function testing indicate that this patient has airflow obstruction. In a young individual with exposure to antigens known to provoke asthma (cat dander, mold), this would raise concern for asthma. However, in addition to the fact that she does not have a response to bronchodilators, the flow–volume curve indicates that she has an obstruction of her upper airway, as there is flattening of the expiratory and inspiratory limbs of the curve (compare to the predicted values). The most appropriate next step in her evaluation would be bronchoscopy to evaluate for a mass lesion or other process narrowing the airway. A CT scan of the head and neck could also be considered to look for a lesion causing external compression. None of the other options listed would be appropriate interventions at this time.

Question 10. B is correct. The key difference in the two sets of tests is that the diffusion capacity for carbon monoxide (D_LCO) is normal for Patient 1 and markedly reduced for Patient 2. Otherwise, both patients have features commonly seen in obstructive lung diseases including a low FEV_1/FVC ratio and increased residual volume (RV). Reductions in the D_LCO are commonly seen in emphysema because enlargement of the airspaces decreases the surface area for gas exchange. Because asthma primarily affects the airways and is not associated with enlargement of the airspaces, the D_LCO is typically normal. In some cases, it may even be increased as a result of increases in lung volume when disease activity is increased.

CHAPTER 5

Question 1. C is correct. The clinical and radiographic findings in this case are consistent with diffuse interstitial pulmonary fibrosis. Because of the increased radial traction on the airways, the FEV_1/FVC percentage is often increased. However, the FEV_1, FVC, and TLC are reduced. Airway resistance when related to lung volume is also reduced.

Question 2. D is correct. The results of the pleural fluid analysis indicate this patient has an exudative effusion: the pleural fluid:serum LDH ratio is greater than 0.6, the pleural fluid:serum protein ratio is greater than 0.5, and the pleural fluid cholesterol is greater than 45 mg/dL. Of the items on the list, the one associated with exudative effusions is cancer metastatic to the pleural space. The other answer choices all cause transudative effusions.

Question 3. E is correct. While progressive dyspnea and a history of smoking raise concern for COPD, the findings pulmonary function testing, including the normal FEV_1/FVC and reduced TLC, are consistent with restrictive rather than obstructive lung disease. The plain chest radiograph shows low lung volumes and bilateral interstitial opacities, while the chest CT shows traction bronchiectasis, honeycombing, and interstitial thickening, all findings consistent with pulmonary fibrosis. Findings on pathologic examination in pulmonary fibrosis include thickening of the alveolar walls and interstitial space with collagen deposition. Enlarged airspaces with loss of alveolar walls are seen in emphysema, while chronic inflammation and hypertrophied mucous glands are seen in chronic bronchitis, and smooth muscle hypertrophy is seen in asthma. Depending on the stage, sarcoidosis could have a similar clinical presentation and imaging findings, but a biopsy would show noncaseating, rather than caseating, granulomas.

Question 4. A is correct. Amyotrophic lateral sclerosis and idiopathic pulmonary fibrosis both cause restrictive pathophysiology. Because pulmonary fibrosis decreases the surface area for gas exchange, a patient with pulmonary fibrosis would have a decreased diffusion capacity for carbon monoxide, whereas the lung parenchyma, surface area for gas exchange, and diffusion capacity would be normal in the patient with amyotrophic lateral sclerosis. The two patients will have similar findings with regard to the FEV_1, FEV_1/FVC ratio, FVC, and total lung capacity.

Question 5. D is correct. This woman has evidence of tension pneumothorax probably due to rupture of a bleb or bullae related to her chronic obstructive pulmonary disease. This is a medical emergency and should be treated with urgent needle decompression of the affected side. None of the other diagnostic tests or interventions would be appropriate.

Question 6. D is correct. The clinical and radiographic information in this case indicates this patient likely has diffuse interstitial fibrosis. On pulmonary function testing, these patients demonstrate decreased FEV_1, FVC, TLC, and DLCO. The FEV_1/FVC ratio is normal and, in some cases, increased.

Question 7. E is correct. The finding of noncaseating granulomas in a patient with bilateral hilar lymphadenopathy is consistent with a diagnosis of sarcoidosis. Although some forms of sarcoidosis, such as asymptomatic hilar lymphadenopathy or Löfgren's syndrome, do not warrant treatment because spontaneous remission is common, this patient has evidence of extrapulmonary disease including eye involvement (anterior uveitis) and cardiac involvement (conduction abnormality), and, as a result, has indications for treatment with systemic corticosteroids. Antifibrotic agents such as pirfenidone are used for idiopathic pulmonary fibrosis, while inhaled antimuscarinic and long-acting β_2-agonists are used in the management of COPD and/or asthma and have no role in the management of sarcoidosis.

Question 8. E is correct. The pulmonary function testing and imaging are consistent with a diagnosis of pulmonary fibrosis. In such cases, ventilation–perfusion mismatch is the primary cause of hypoxemia at rest. Although the alveolar–capillary barrier is thickened and diffusion of oxygen across the barrier is slower, under resting conditions, there is still enough time for full equilibration between the alveolar and pulmonary capillary P_{O_2}. As a result, diffusion impairment does not contribute significantly to resting hypoxemia compared to ventilation–perfusion mismatch. Hypoventilation is not typically present until very late stages of pulmonary fibrosis. In fact, many patients have a respiratory alkalosis due to the ventilatory response to hypoxemia. An abnormally small rise in cardiac output may play a role in worsening hypoxemia with exercise but decreased cardiac output is not typically present at rest and, therefore, does not contribute to hypoxemia.

Question 9. C is correct. The pulmonary function tests and chest radiograph suggest the patient has restrictive physiology due to a diffuse parenchymal lung disease. The fact that she owns two pet cockatiels would raise concern for hypersensitivity pneumonitis. Due to stimulation of peripheral chemoreceptors by hypoxemia and stimulation of other receptors within the lung, she will likely have respiratory alkalosis. Because her symptoms have been going on for many months, there has been adequate time for renal compensation, so she should have a compensated rather than an acute respiratory alkalosis. Respiratory acidosis typically only occurs in the very late stages of diffuse parenchymal lung diseases.

Question 10. A is correct. The pulmonary function tests show evidence of restrictive lung disease. The normal diffusion capacity for carbon monoxide makes hypersensitivity pneumonitis, idiopathic pulmonary fibrosis, and sarcoidosis unlikely as the cause. The maximum inspiratory and expiratory pressure measurements provide information about muscle strength. The fact that the inspiratory muscle strength is very low, while the expiratory muscle strength is normal suggests this patient could have isolated diaphragmatic weakness, as a diffuse neuromuscular disease like muscular dystrophy would cause weakness of the expiratory and inspiratory muscles.

CHAPTER 6

Question 1. B is correct. The sudden onset of dyspnea and chest pain following a period of prolonged immobility as well as the finding of asymmetric leg edema on examination raises concern for pulmonary embolism. The most appropriate diagnostic test is a contrast-enhanced CT scan of the chest. Pulmonary angiography is the gold standard for diagnosis of pulmonary embolism but is very invasive and would not be done before a CT scan. The other choices would not yield the correct diagnosis in this case.

Question 2. B is correct. This patient has elevated pulmonary artery pressure in the setting of pulmonary edema due to left heart failure. Left ventricular failure leads to increased left ventricular end-diastolic and left atrial pressure, which contributes to increased pulmonary artery pressure. Without other evidence of sarcoidosis, granulomatous inflammation of the arterioles would not be expected. Increased pulmonary blood flow occurs with ventricular septal defects or patent ductus arteriosus but would not be expected in left ventricular failure. Her history is not consistent with either idiopathic pulmonary arterial hypertension, which would cause structural changes in the arterioles, or recurrent thromboembolism.

Question 3. D is correct. This individual likely has high altitude pulmonary edema (HAPE), which develops as a result of exaggerated hypoxic pulmonary vasoconstriction. The arteriolar constriction is uneven and, as a result, regions of the capillary bed that are not protected from the high pressure develop the ultrastructural changes of stress failure. Left ventricular function and, therefore, left atrial pressure are normal in HAPE, while colloid osmotic pressure, and interstitial pressure are unaffected. Endotoxin-mediated increases in capillary permeability are seen in sepsis rather than at high altitude.

Question 4. D is correct. This patient with very severe COPD is now presenting with signs of cor pulmonale including increased jugular venous distention, weight gain, and bilateral leg edema and characteristic changes on electrocardiography. The most appropriate test to confirm this diagnosis would be echocardiography. Since he is known to have COPD, spirometry would not provide further useful information. Duplex ultrasonography and contrast-enhanced CT are not indicated, as the suspicion for venous thromboembolism is low. Bronchoscopy would not be helpful in the evaluation of cor pulmonale.

Question 5. A is correct. Several aspects of this patient's presentation suggest he may have hereditary hemorrhagic telangiectasia (HHT). In addition to the presence of telangiectasias on examination, he has both platypnea (dyspnea that is worse in the upright position) and orthodeoxia (decrease in oxygen saturation when in the upright position) and evidence of a significant shunt on his arterial blood gas studies (the P_{O_2} only rises to 300 mm Hg while breathing an inspired oxygen fraction of 1.0). A family history of mucocutaneous bleeding is also consistent with this diagnosis. These patients commonly develop pulmonary arteriovenous malformations (AVMs). Because these large, abnormal communications between the pulmonary arteries and pulmonary veins bypass the normal filter function of the pulmonary capillary network, individuals with HHT are at risk for strokes and intracerebral abscess.

Question 6. C is correct. The clinical presentation is most consistent with pulmonary edema due to decompensated heart failure. The chest radiograph shows a large heart with bilateral alveolar opacities, while the physical examination demonstrates several findings seen with worsening heart failure including increased jugular venous pulsation, crackles on lung examination, and pitting lower extremity edema. Airway resistance is typically increased in pulmonary edema due to multiple factors including peribronchial cuffing from interstitial edema, reflex bronchoconstriction due to stimulation of irritant receptors in the bronchial walls and, in some cases, edema fluid in the airways. Lung compliance is reduced, while the elastic recoil of the lung is increased. Closing volume may increase as a result of the increased airways resistance. The diffusing capacity for carbon monoxide would be decreased.

Question 7. D is correct. The image from the CT scan shows filling defects in both the left and right main pulmonary arteries, consistent with pulmonary embolism. Intimal injury following his hip fracture as well as immobility in the postoperative period were likely the predisposing factors to this problem. Hypoxemia develops in pulmonary embolism largely due to ventilation–perfusion inequality with one of the major causes being redistribution of blood flow to nonembolized areas of the lung; increased perfusion of these areas without significant changes in ventilation lowers the ventilation–perfusion ratios of those units. The fact that the arterial P_{CO_2} is normal tells us that alveolar ventilation is appropriate for the level of CO_2 production (i.e., there is no hypoventilation). Airway secretions are not increased in pulmonary embolism, nor is the alveolar–capillary barrier affected. Significant increases in pulmonary artery pressure can open the foramen ovale, but this leads to right-to-left, rather than left-to-right, shunt.

Question 8. D is correct. This patient has pulmonary hypertension (mean pulmonary artery pressure greater than 25 mm Hg) associated with increased pulmonary vascular resistance (PVR). Of the items on the list, the one most likely to cause this clinical picture, including the right heart catheterization data, is pulmonary arterial hypertension in which intimal thickening, medial hypertrophy, and plexiform arteriopathy narrow pulmonary arterioles and increase PVR. Advanced chronic obstructive pulmonary disease (COPD) can also cause pulmonary hypertension, but the normal FEV_1/ FVC ratio rules this as a cause. Mitral stenosis is unlikely given the normal pulmonary artery occlusion pressure, a marker of left atrial pressure. Ventricular septal defects cause pulmonary hypertension due to increased pulmonary blood flow rather than high vascular resistance, although this can be seen due to structural remodeling over time. This is unlikely given the lack of a prior past medical history and a murmur on examination. Arteriovenous malformations are large abnormal vascular communications between branches of the pulmonary arteries and veins and, as such, typically lower pulmonary vascular resistance.

Question 9. E is correct. This patient developed pulmonary edema 4 days following a myocardial infarction. Given the new murmur and the findings on echocardiography, this is most likely due to acute mitral regurgitation, an uncommon but severe complication of myocardial infarction resulting from injury to the papillary muscles. As a result of the acute valvular dysfunction, there is a large increase in both left atrial and pulmonary venous pressure, which subsequently causes a significant rise in pulmonary capillary hydrostatic pressure. Decreased interstitial and increased pulmonary capillary colloid osmotic pressure would actually decrease the likelihood of edema formation, as would increased interstitial hydrostatic pressure. None of these factors would play a role in this situation. Increased lymphatic drainage would also decrease the likelihood of pulmonary edema and is one of the things that helps prevent edema in patients in whom mitral regurgitation develops over a longer period of time compared to the abrupt onset seen in this case scenario.

CHAPTER 7

Question 1. A is correct. Many features of this patient's case suggest he has diffuse pulmonary fibrosis. Given that he worked with insulation in the shipyards and has calcified pleural plaques on his chest radiograph, this is most likely due to asbestosis. His spirometry is not consistent with chronic obstructive pulmonary disease, and his chest radiograph and exposure history are not compatible with berylliosis, coal worker's pneumoconiosis or silicosis.

Question 2. B is correct. The diagnosis of pneumocystis pneumonia should always prompt evaluation for underlying immunosuppression, in particular human immunodeficiency virus (HIV) as it is uncommon in immunocompetent individuals. Sweat chloride testing is used to evaluate for cystic fibrosis. Individuals living with HIV at increased risk for TB, but skin testing would not be helpful in this situation. Spirometry and echocardiography would not be useful.

Question 3. C is correct. The majority of particles released as part of the accident are larger than 10 μm in diameter. Large particles (greater than 20 μm) are very likely to be removed by the nose or impact the airway mucosa in the nasopharynx. Medium-size particles (1 to 5 μm) will deposit by sedimentation in the terminal and respiratory bronchioles, while very small particles (less than 0.1 μm in diameter) may deposit by diffusion in the small airways and alveoli.

Question 4. E is correct. The presence of fever, dyspnea, and productive cough in conjunction with a focal opacity on chest radiography suggests that this patient has pneumonia. In pneumonia, the lung affected by the disease is not ventilated, and, if it is perfused, the resulting shunt can cause hypoxemia. Carbon dioxide retention (i.e., hypoventilation) is unlikely in most patients because of increased ventilation to other parts of the lung. While diffusion may be slower due to the presence of an inflammatory exudate in the alveolar space, this does not contribute to hypoxemia due to the large reserve of time available for diffusion. Hypoxic vasoconstriction protects against hypoxemia by diverting blood flow from poorly or unventilated areas. Decreased cardiac output can contribute to hypoxemia by decreasing the mixed venous P_{O_2}, but the fact that the patient is normotensive, has a normal mental status, and appears warm and well perfused suggests that his cardiac output is normal.

Question 5. B is correct. Recurrent sinopulmonary infections, dilated, thickened airways on chest imaging suggestive of bronchiectasis and the finding of the ΔF508 mutation indicate this child has cystic fibrosis (CF). Patients with CF suffer from impaired mucous clearance and obstruction of airways and ducts. One of the main reasons for this is decreased sodium efflux from the respiratory epithelium, which reduces hydration of the mucous layer surrounding the cilia. As a result, the cilia do not beat properly and are ineffective at helping to clear mucous out of the airways. This predisposes to recurrent infections and ongoing airway inflammation. None of the other answer choices play a role in CF.

Question 6. E is correct. The molecules in a gas are too small to impact or sediment and, instead, deposit largely as a result of diffusion. Deposition by diffusion occurs primarily in the small airways and alveoli. As a result, of the items on the list, the most likely location at which the gas will deposit is the respiratory bronchioles. Large particles would get caught in the nasal passages or more proximal airways depending on their size.

Question 7. E is correct. The patient has a mixed obstructive–restrictive pattern on pulmonary function testing as indicated by the fact that both the FEV_1/FVC ratio and the total lung capacity are reduced. The chest radiograph shows prominent, bilateral confluent opacities, similar to those seen in progressive massive fibrosis. The fact that the patient spent a long time working as a sandblaster suggests that his clinical findings are most likely related to silicosis. Patients with silicosis are at increased risk for pulmonary tuberculosis. The reasons for the increased risk are not entirely clear, but may relate to effects of silica on macrophage function.

Question 8. B is correct. This patient has a mass that is partially obstructing the right main bronchus. The extensive smoking history and recent weight loss suggest this mass could be a lung cancer. Partial obstruction of a large bronchus can cause an obstructive pattern on pulmonary function testing, the hallmark of which is a reduced FEV_1/FVC ratio. Decreased total lung capacity, residual volume, and closing volume can be seen in restrictive processes due to parenchymal lung disease. Large pleural effusions in lung cancer can cause restrictive pathophysiology, but there is no evidence of such an effusion on her chest imaging. There is no reason to suspect this patient would have an increased diffusing capacity for carbon monoxide.

CHAPTER 8

Question 1. C is correct. Excessive supplemental oxygen administration in patients with severe COPD and CO_2 retention can paradoxically worsen their hypercapnia. This occurs for several reasons. An important cause of this is release of hypoxic vasoconstriction in poorly ventilated areas of lung as a result of the increased alveolar P_{O_2}. This increases blood flow to poorly ventilated areas, which impairs CO_2 elimination and exaggerates the CO_2 retention. In addition, ventilatory drive in this patient is augmented by hypoxemia. By raising the arterial P_{O_2} too high, this added drive to ventilation is removed; ventilation decreases and P_{CO_2} increases. This was not one of the answer choices. The other choices are incorrect.

Question 2. D is correct. An exacerbation of chronic obstructive pulmonary disease often causes an increase in arterial P_{CO_2} and therefore respiratory acidosis. The other choices are incorrect. Mechanical ventilation and administration of antibiotics will reduce the tendency to CO_2 retention. The pH will be low in the acute phase of an exacerbation but will return toward normal due to renal retention of bicarbonate (metabolic compensation).

Question 3. C is correct. This patient has developed the acute respiratory distress syndrome (ARDS). Less than 7 days after a significant trauma, he has severe hypoxemic respiratory failure with diffuse bilateral opacities in the absence of cardiac dysfunction. Severe hypoxemia is common in ARDS and typically is due to ventilation–perfusion mismatch and, in particular, marked increases in blood flow to low $\dot{V}_A/\dot{Q}$ alveoli, as well as shunt. Lung elastic recoil is actually increased in ARDS due to increased surface tension forces related to alveolar edema and exudate. Both functional residual capacity and lung compliance are reduced as a result of this change in elastic recoil. The airways are not significantly affected by ARDS, and, as a result, airways resistance is not typically increased, although some increase in resistance can be seen when patients develop airway secretions.

Question 4. E is correct. The development of hypoxemic respiratory failure with diffuse opacities shortly after premature birth usually results from the neonatal respiratory distress syndrome due to insufficient pulmonary surfactant. In addition to supportive care, appropriate treatment includes administration of surfactant by the inhalational route. Bronchodilators would not be useful in this situation since the pathophysiology is related to extensive alveolar atelectasis. Diuretics such as furosemide and digoxin would also not be of use as the infant is not in heart failure.

Question 5. E is correct. An acute exacerbation of chronic obstructive pulmonary disease in a patient with severe COPD typically causes worsening of ventilation–perfusion matching. The other choices are incorrect. COPD exacerbations increase the airway resistance; the arterial pH typically falls because of worsening respiratory acidosis, and the alveolar–arterial P_{O_2} difference increases.

Question 6. B is correct. This patient presented with acute hypoxemic respiratory failure and has evidence of tissue hypoxia including confusion, cool mottled distal extremities, and an increased lactate concentration. The findings on physical examination (displaced point of maximal impulse and lower extremity edema), chest radiograph, and echocardiogram all suggest this patient has pulmonary edema due to heart failure. In addition to providing supplemental oxygen, tissue oxygen delivery can be increased by improving cardiac output with the use of the inotrope dobutamine. A red blood cell transfusion is not indicated since she not anemic. Antibiotics are not indicated as there is no evidence of pneumonia (afebrile, normal white blood cell count, no focal opacity on chest imaging). Surfactant is only administered in neonatal respiratory distress syndrome, while noninvasive positive pressure ventilation is not indicated because she does not have evidence of hypoventilation.

Question 7. B is correct. This patient has acute respiratory failure due to an opiate overdose. The increased arterial P_{CO_2} on his arterial blood gas indicates that his hypoxemia is due to hypoventilation. Using the alveolar gas equation, we can determine the ideal alveolar P_{O_2}, which, assuming R = 0.8, turns out to be 66 mm Hg. The alveolar arterial P_{O_2} difference, therefore, is 10 mm Hg. This is a normal value, which indicates that neither shunt nor ventilation–perfusion inequality is contributing to his hypoxemia. This is a case of pure hypoventilation. Even though the alveolar P_{O_2} is low and the gradient for diffusion across the alveolar–capillary barrier is reduced, there is still adequate time for diffusion and diffusion impairment does not contribute to hypoxemia in this case.

Question 8. C is correct. A several day history of fever, productive cough, and dyspnea with focal findings on examination and chest radiography and a leukocytosis on laboratory studies is consistent with a diagnosis of pneumonia. The causes of hypoxemia in pneumonia are shunt and ventilation–perfusion inequality. Despite impaired ventilation to the affected part of the lung, these patients rarely develop hypercapnia because increased ventilation leads to elimination of carbon dioxide from noninvolved areas of the lung. Instead, it is more common to see either a normal or low arterial P_{CO_2} on an arterial blood gas. This would correspond to point C on the O_2–CO_2 diagram.

CHAPTER 9

Question 1. E is correct. Fifty percent oxygen raises the inspired P_{O_2} to about 350 mm Hg from its normal value of about 150 mm Hg. Therefore, if the P_{CO_2} does not change, we can expect the alveolar P_{O_2} to rise by approximately 200 mm Hg. Because this patient's hypoxemia is due to hypoventilation and there is no ventilation–perfusion inequality, the alveolar–arterial P_{O_2} difference should remain small. As a result, the arterial P_{O_2} should also increase by about 200 mm Hg.

Question 2. C is correct. The arterial P_{O_2} will rise because of the oxygen dissolved in the nonshunted blood. However, it cannot possibly rise to 600 mm Hg because of the 20% right-to-left shunt. Therefore, the only possible correct choices are B and C. Figure 9.3 and the accompanying text shows that the P_{O_2} should increase by more than 10 mm Hg. It is a common misperception that shunt does not respond at all to supplemental oxygen. When shunt contributes to hypoxemia, the P_{O_2} will rise with supplemental oxygen administration, but the increase is not as large as it would be if hypoventilation, diffusion impairment, or ventilation–perfusion mismatch were the cause of hypoxemia. Instead, the size of the response varies based on the magnitude of the right-to-left shunt.

Question 3. A is correct. In addition to having a much higher affinity for hemoglobin than oxygen and, as a result, outcompeting oxygen for the hemoglobin-binding sites, carbon monoxide increases the oxygen affinity of the hemoglobin. This is represented by a decrease in the P_{50} for hemoglobin. The other choices are incorrect. The arterial oxygen content should go down due to reduction in the amount of oxygen bound to hemoglobin. The mixed venous P_{O_2} goes down due to increased tissue oxygen extraction in response to the decreased oxygen delivery. Arterial pH may fall if the decrease in oxygen delivery causes a lactic acidosis. The 2,3-DPG concentration should not decrease in this situation.

Question 4. C is correct. The solubility of oxygen is 0.003 mL/100 mL blood/mm Hg. A pressure of 3 atmospheres is equivalent to 2,280 mm Hg so that with an inspired concentration of 100%, we can expect the inspired P_{O_2} to rise to more than 2,000 mm Hg. Therefore, the amount of dissolved oxygen will be approximately 6 mL/100 mL.

Question 5. A is correct. The significant increase in arterial P_{O_2} and $S_{P_{O_2}}$ following supplemental oxygen administration decreases peripheral chemoreceptor stimulation, leading to decreased minute and alveolar ventilation and a rise in the arterial P_{CO_2}. Because alveolar P_{O_2} increases with supplemental oxygen administration, ventilation–perfusion matching will worsen rather than improve. The hemoglobin oxygen dissociation curve shifts to the right due to the increase in P_{CO_2} but does not cause the hypercarbia. Increased hemoglobin–oxygen saturation decreases formation of carbamino groups on the hemoglobin chains, while the rise in arterial P_{CO_2} causes a decrease in arterial pH.

Question 6. B is correct. When high concentrations of oxygen are administered, lung units with low ventilation–perfusion ratios may deliver oxygen into the blood faster than it enters by ventilation. The units, therefore, collapse. The other choices are incorrect. Pulmonary surfactant is not inactivated. Oxygen toxicity causes alveolar edema, but this is not the mechanism of alveolar collapse. Interstitial edema can develop around small airways, but this does not lead to increased shunt. Similarly, inflammatory changes and smooth muscle contraction in the airways may occur but would not increase the shunt fraction.

Question 7. C is correct. When this patient was placed on mechanical ventilation with an inspired oxygen fraction of 1.0, the arterial P_{O_2} only rose to 100 mm Hg. This indicates that shunt is the primary cause of hypoxemia, as the arterial P_{O_2} would have increased to nearly 600 mm Hg when breathing an inspired oxygen fraction of 1.0 if hypoxemia was due to diffusion impairment, hypoventilation, or ventilation–perfusion inequality. Ventilation–perfusion inequality may be contributing to hypoxemia in this patient, but the fact that the alveolar–arterial P_{O_2} difference is so large on an inspired oxygen fraction of 1.0 suggests shunt is the primary cause. The fact that the arterial P_{CO_2} is below 40 is another reason why hypoxemia cannot be attributed to hypoventilation in this case.

Question 8. D is correct. The mixed venous oxygen concentration is a function of the arterial oxygen content, tissue oxygen consumption ($\dot{V}O_2$), and cardiac output (see Equation 9.2). Following administration of dobutamine, the cardiac output increased, and there was a small increase in the arterial P_{O_2}. As a result, oxygen delivery to the tissues increases. Tissue oxygen extraction falls, thereby leading to an increase in the mixed venous oxygen concentration. Improved tissue oxygen delivery should not lead to lactic acidosis and a decrease in serum pH. Tissue oxygen consumption should not change in this situation.

Question 9. A is correct. This patient is hypoxemic and requires supplemental oxygen. Although there are typically several options for providing oxygen, because she has a high inspiratory flow rate, the regular nasal cannula, and the simple, venturi, and nonrebreather masks may not deliver a predictable inspired oxygen concentration. The flow of gas to these delivery devices is limited, and, as a result, there is considerable entrainment of ambient air in patients with a high inspiratory flow rate. By delivering gas at flow rates as high as 60 L/min, a high-flow nasal cannula limits the entrainment of ambient air, thereby yielding a more predictable increase in the inspired oxygen concentration.

CHAPTER 10

Question 1. C is correct. When the P_{O_2} does not rise significantly in patients with ARDS following a large increase in the F_IO_2, the appropriate intervention is to increase the positive end-expiratory pressure (PEEP). Increasing the tidal volume and/or rate would increase minute ventilation, but this would likely not translate to an increase in the arterial P_{O_2} due to the severe ventilation–perfusion mismatch and shunt. Increasing the flow rate would prolong the expiratory phase but would not affect oxygenation, while changing to pressure control ventilation would also have no effect on oxygenation if the same F_IO_2 and PEEP were used.

Question 2. A is correct. The patient's blood pressure likely fell due to a decrease in venous return that occurred with initiation of positive pressure ventilation. This was likely exacerbated by the fact that she was volume depleted due to her hemorrhagic shock. Tension pneumothorax can cause hypotension, but this is unlikely given that she has bilateral breath sounds, and her trachea is in the midline position. Hypercarbia, resorption atelectasis, and right mainstem intubation would not affect her blood pressure.

Question 3. C is correct. The description provided corresponds to the pressure control mode of mechanical ventilation. Pressure support also involves raising the inspiratory pressure a preset amount above the set PEEP, but there is no set respiratory rate and inspiratory pressure ceases when flow decreases sufficiently rather than after a prespecified time period. Volume control involves administering a preset volume rather than an inspiratory pressure. The ventilator does not change airway pressure during inhalation or exhalation in continuous positive airway pressure. High-frequency ventilation involves using very small tidal volumes (50 to 150 mL) at a very high frequency.

Question 4. C is correct. If the total ventilation is kept constant, the alveolar ventilation can be raised by increasing the tidal volume. This raises the ratio of alveolar ventilation to total ventilation, but of course reduces the respiratory frequency. The other choices are incorrect. Reducing the FRC will not directly affect ventilation, although it may result in atelectatic areas. Increasing the respiratory frequency necessarily means lowering the tidal volume, and thus reducing the ratio of alveolar ventilation to total ventilation. Reducing the resistance of the airways, if that can be done, will not change alveolar ventilation. Finally, adding oxygen to the inspired gas also does not change alveolar ventilation.

Question 5. A is correct. PEEP can be an effective tool for increasing the arterial P_{O_2} when patients fail to respond to increases in the inspired oxygen fraction due to large shunts. At the same time, the increase in alveolar pressure can compress the pulmonary capillaries, which tends to divert blood flow away from ventilated regions causing either high ventilation–perfusion ratios or dead space. Capillary compression leads to an increase in pulmonary vascular resistance, while the increase in lung volume increases radial traction on the airways and lowers airway resistance. Increased PEEP tends to decrease venous return.

Question 6. C is correct. This patient has obstructive lung disease, as evidenced by the pulmonary function test results performed several weeks earlier. He is now presenting with an exacerbation of his chronic obstructive pulmonary disease (COPD) as evidenced by his increasing dyspnea and the findings on examination and chest radiography. All of the interventions in the list of answer choices would improve his hypoxemia. However, the arterial blood gas reveals that the patient has an acute respiratory acidosis. As a result, it is important to provide ventilatory support and address his impaired respiratory mechanics. This can only be done with noninvasive positive pressure ventilation or invasive mechanical ventilation. In patients with COPD, it is appropriate to begin with noninvasive positive pressure ventilation before intubating the patient and initiating invasive mechanical ventilation.

Question 7. D is correct. When an endotracheal tube is inserted too deep in the airway, the tip will typically reside in the right mainstem bronchus. This occurs because of the differences in the angles at which the right and left mainstem bronchi branch off the trachea. Overinsertion of the tube impairs ventilation to the left lung. Quite often, ventilation is reduced to the right upper lobe as well because the tip of the tube lies distal to the bronchus serving this lobe. As a result, there can be atelectasis of both the left lung and the right upper lobe. Decreased venous return is unlikely on this level of PEEP and would not cause the findings on chest radiography. Ventilator-induced lung injury is unlikely on a tidal volume of 8 mL/kg and would not cause focal atelectasis. Administration of a high inspired oxygen fraction can cause resorption atelectasis when airways are occluded, but it would not develop this quickly, nor would it cause the pattern of atelectasis seen on the chest radiograph. A respiratory alkalosis, if present, would not lead to atelectasis.

Question 8. A is correct. PEEP is often used to improve oxygenation in patients receiving invasive mechanical ventilation. Despite the small increase in the arterial P_{O_2}, the patient's mixed venous oxygen content fell from 14 to 12 mL O_2/100 mL, suggesting that tissue oxygen delivery must have decreased. Given that the hemoglobin concentration remained constant, the fall in oxygen delivery must be the result of a decrease in cardiac output, which can happen following increases in PEEP due to reductions in venous return. Pulmonary vascular resistance can increase with PEEP due to compression of pulmonary capillaries. Airway resistance typically decreases due to increased radial traction due to the increase in lung volume. Increases in PEEP can cause barotrauma, but pneumomediastinum does not typically impair venous return.

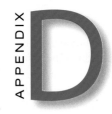
ANSWERS TO QUESTIONS IN CLINICAL VIGNETTES

CHAPTER 1

The FEV_1 is decreased while the FVC is within the normal range. The decreased FEV_1/FVC ratio indicates that the patient has airflow obstruction. The FEV_1 improves by 0.2 L (7% change), while the FVC is unchanged following administration of a short-acting bronchodilator indicating the patient does not meet criteria for a bronchodilator response (increase in FEV_1 or FVC by 200 mL and 12% from prebronchodilator values). The presence of airflow obstruction in a young individual typically raises concern for asthma, but the presence of flattening of both the inspiratory and expiratory limb of the flow–volume loop strongly suggests that the airflow obstruction is due to something other than asthma. In particular, this pattern is consistent with a fixed upper airway obstruction. This patient was subsequently sent for a CT scan of the chest, which demonstrated extensive lymphadenopathy compressing the intrathoracic trachea. Surgical biopsy later confirmed that this was due to lymphoma.

CHAPTER 2

Spirometry performed in clinic 2 weeks ago demonstrates severe airflow obstruction with air trapping (increased RV) but no hyperinflation or bronchodilator response. In a patient with a long history of tobacco use, these findings are consistent with those seen in chronic obstructive pulmonary disease (COPD). Her increased dyspnea along with a change in the frequency of her cough and a change in the character of her sputum production suggest that she has a COPD exacerbation. On examination, this typically causes diffuse expiratory wheezes, a prolonged expiratory phase, and hyperresonant lung fields. The decreased diffusion capacity for carbon monoxide indicates that the surface area for gas exchange is decreased. When this occurs in the setting of airflow obstruction, it suggests that the patient has underlying emphysema.

The arterial blood gas demonstrates an acute respiratory acidosis, a common finding in COPD exacerbations. The increased arterial P_{CO_2} and the increased alveolar–arterial P_{O_2} difference (27 mm Hg) are caused by increased ventilation–perfusion inequality. By raising airway pressure on inhalation, noninvasive ventilation through a tight-fitting mask will increase her total and alveolar ventilation and, as a result, decrease her arterial P_{CO_2}.

CHAPTER 3

This patient has hypersensitivity pneumonitis due to her pet cockatiel. Her pulmonary function tests demonstrate restrictive pathophysiology. The decreased diffusion capacity for carbon monoxide indicates that the restriction is due to an intraparenchymal process. FRC, which is due to the balance between lung and chest recoil, decreases due to increased lung recoil. RV will likely be low because lung compliance is reduced, and the interstitial lung disease leads to increased radial traction on her airways, which allows more air to exit the lungs on exhalation. The compliance of her lungs will decrease as a result of her parenchymal process, causing the pressure–volume curve for her lungs to shift down and to the right and have a lower slope than in a healthy individual. While airway resistance is increased in obstructive lung diseases, in a diffuse interstitial process, the airways are unaffected and resistance should be normal. In fact, if radial traction on the airways increases as a result of her disease, then airway resistance at any lung volume would be lower than that in a healthy individual. During a cardiopulmonary exercise test, her arterial P_{O_2} would be expected to decrease due to increased ventilation–perfusion mismatch and possibly some diffusion impairment. Mixed venous P_{O_2} also decreases in exercise due to reduced cardiac output, and this will also contribute to the development of hypoxemia in the setting of ventilation–perfusion inequality.

CHAPTER 4

This patient is having an acute asthma exacerbation. In such cases, the functional residual capacity and residual volume are increased compared to when a patient is in his or her normal healthy state. The hyperinflation seen on chest radiography would fit with such findings. The increased RV is due to premature airway closure on exhalation, while the cause of the increased FRC is not fully understood. Even though patients with asthma exacerbations are having airflow obstruction on exhalation, they commonly report that they have difficulty with inhalation. This is because air trapping and hyperinflation create a mechanical disadvantage. One particular problem is the flattening of the diaphragm, which impairs its contractile efficiency. Hypoxemia in these situations is primarily due to ventilation–perfusion inequality, although in severe cases, shunt may contribute if considerable mucous plugging of airways is present. Despite the fact that he is having significant difficulty breathing, the arterial P_{CO_2} is typically low during an asthma exacerbation due to increased ventilation resulting from stimulation of the peripheral chemoreceptors by hypoxemia or stimulation of intrapulmonary receptors. The finding of a rising arterial P_{CO_2} during an asthma exacerbation is an ominous finding and suggests the patient is developing respiratory failure due to ventilatory muscle fatigue and increasing ventilation–perfusion inequality. Treatment for an asthma exacerbation includes supplemental oxygen, systemic corticosteroids, and nebulized β_2-agonists. If he fails to improve and manifests evidence of respiratory failure, he may require intubation and mechanical ventilation.

CHAPTER 5

The finding of noncaseating granulomas on transbronchial biopsy indicates that this patient has sarcoidosis. In addition to bilateral hilar lymphadenopathy, her chest radiograph demonstrates diffuse bilateral reticular lung opacities. Based on this finding as well as the fact that her FEV_1 and FVC are reduced with a normal FEV_1/FVC ratio, she will likely have a restrictive pathophysiology and, therefore, a low TLC. We would also anticipate from the radiographic findings that her surface area for gas exchange is abnormal, and therefore, her diffusing capacity for carbon monoxide will be low. Because of the changes in her lung parenchyma, her lung compliance will be low, and therefore, the pressure–volume curve will be shifted down and to the right with a lower slope than in a healthy individual. On an arterial blood sample, she will either have normal acid–base status or a compensated respiratory alkalosis. The latter finding can develop if the patient has hyperventilation due to hypoxemia and subsequent stimulation of the peripheral chemoreceptors and/or stimulation of intrapulmonary receptors. If her parenchymal lung disease worsens significantly despite treatment, she may ultimately develop respiratory failure and progressive hypercarbia. This would lead to a compensated respiratory acidosis. With exercise, her arterial P_{O_2} will likely decrease and the alveolar–arterial P_{O_2} difference will widen as a result of increased ventilation–perfusion inequality due to the extensive parenchymal lung disease.

CHAPTER 6

The acute onset of chest pain, dyspnea, and hypoxemia following repair of pelvic or long-bone fractures should always raise concern for pulmonary embolism. The diagnosis was confirmed in this case by the identification of a filling defect on the CT pulmonary angiogram. The major risk factor for pulmonary embolism in this case was vascular injury related to her pelvic fracture and its surgical repair. A lack of mobility following her operation may also have contributed. In such settings, unfractionated or low molecular weight heparin is often given on a prophylactic basis to prevent this problem. The echocardiography might show an elevation in pulmonary artery pressure due to obstruction to blood flow, but this depends on the size of the embolus. Small emboli will have little effect, but larger emboli are more likely to do so. Pulmonary embolism increases the physiologic dead space, but her arterial P_{CO_2} remained normal because she was able to increase her total ventilation. In some cases, the hypoxemia, severe pain, and anxiety following pulmonary embolism cause patients to raise their total ventilation even more, in which case a low P_{CO_2} may be seen. Hypoxemia develops primarily as a result of ventilation–perfusion inequality that develops due to redistribution of blood flow to the nonembolized regions of the lung.

CHAPTER 7

This patient has cystic fibrosis, a multisystem disease that develops due to one of a variety of mutations affecting the cystic fibrosis transmembrane regulator (CFTR). These defects lead to alterations in sodium and chloride transport, which impair mucous clearance and lead to plugging of airways as well as ducts in other organs. Decreased mucociliary transport subsequently leads to persistent inflammation and infection in the airways, which, overtime, contributes to the development of bronchiectasis and airflow obstruction. The tubular structures seen in the upper lung zones are dilated airways and are indicative of the presence of bronchiectasis. Increased airway secretions typically lead to findings of airflow obstruction on pulmonary function testing including decreased $FEF_{25\%-75\%}$, increased RV/TLC ratio, and decreased FEV_1/FVC. While hyperinflation can lead to a high TLC, some patients eventually develop a mixed obstructive–restrictive defect as the TLC declines due to extensive scarring. Airway clearance measures such as regular exercise, chest physiotherapy, flutter devices, and percussion vests as well as medications such as inhaled DNAase and hypertonic saline are critical for the long-term health of these patients as they help remove secretions from the airways and mitigate the ongoing inflammation and infection that contribute to disease progression. Even with effective treatment, some patients are prone to development of hemoptysis as the ongoing inflammation can erode into the hypertrophied bronchial circulation feeding the airway mucosa. Because the bronchial circulation is perfused under systemic pressure, the volume of expectorated blood can reach life-threatening levels.

CHAPTER 8

This patient has developed the acute respiratory distress syndrome (ARDS) as a consequence of her severe pancreatitis. She developed respiratory failure within 7 days of the pancreatitis, has severe hypoxemia with a low Pa_{O_2}/F_IO_2 ratio, and has diffuse bilateral opacities on chest imaging, and there is no evidence this is related to left heart dysfunction. Due to the extensive injury to the lung, respiratory system compliance is markedly reduced and the pressure–volume curve is shifted downward and to the right. One manifestation of this will be that the mechanical ventilator will require high pressures to inflate her lung with each breath. The functional residual capacity is decreased, likely due to exaggeration of surface tension forces by the alveolar edema and exudate. The fact that her arterial P_{O_2} is only 66 mm Hg while she is receiving 100% oxygen indicates that shunt is the primary cause of her hypoxemia. This is due to the fact that blood continues to flow by alveoli that are filled with edema and exudate and, as a result, do not receive any ventilation. Despite the severe ventilation–perfusion inequality and shunt, the P_{CO_2} may be normal or even low as it is with this patient. This is because the large volume of gas delivered to the alveoli is sufficient to keep the arterial P_{CO_2} normal but not the arterial P_{O_2} in the presence of severe ventilation–perfusion inequality. Some patients with ARDS do develop hypercarbia.

CHAPTER 9

This patient has a left lower lobe pneumonia associated with significant hypoxemia. The fact that the arterial P_{O_2} only increases from 55 to 62 mm Hg while breathing an F_IO_2 of 1.0 indicates that shunt is the primary cause of hypoxemia. Blood continues to perfuse alveoli that are unventilated because they are filled with a neutrophilic exudate. Fever causes a rightward shift in the hemoglobin–oxygen dissociation curve (increased P50) such that any given arterial P_{O_2}, the oxygen saturation is lower. If the cardiac output does not increase sufficiently to compensate for the decrease in saturation, tissue oxygen delivery will decrease. Coupled with the increase in oxygen consumption due to infection and fever, this decrease in oxygen delivery will lead to increased tissue oxygen extraction and a fall in the oxygen content of mixed venous blood. This is a disadvantage from the standpoint of his arterial oxygenation as the oxygen-depleted mixed venous blood cannot pick up oxygen as it traverses the capillary network in the left lower lobe. When oxygenation does not improve despite a high inspired oxygen fraction on mechanical ventilation, positive end-expiratory pressure (PEEP) can be increased to address the hypoxemia (see Chapter 10). This is often not effective in focal processes such as lobar pneumonia, however. One other consideration for this patient would be to give him a blood transfusion, as improving his hemoglobin concentration would increase tissue oxygen delivery and raise the oxygen content of the mixed venous blood. In the setting of shunt, such improvements in mixed venous oxygen content can improve arterial oxygen content.

CHAPTER 10

This patient was intubated for respiratory failure due to severe pneumonia. The fact that she had a high arterial P_{CO_2} prior to intubation indicates that she had inadequate alveolar ventilation in addition to her severe hypoxemia. With initiation of volume control ventilation, which provides a guaranteed level of minute ventilation, she is now receiving sufficient alveolar ventilation to eliminate the carbon dioxide produced in her tissues and the arterial P_{CO_2} decreases. Even though her alveolar ventilation increased, it does not increase by the same amount as total ventilation because mechanical ventilation will increase the volume of both the alveolar and anatomic dead spaces. One cause of this is that the increase in lung volume and application of PEEP increase radial traction on the airways increasing anatomic dead space. Increased airway pressure can also compress alveolar capillaries and divert blood flow away from ventilated regions, thereby causing areas of high ventilation–perfusion ratio or even no perfusion at all.

Her chest radiograph following intubation revealed diffuse bilateral opacities, which, along with her severe hypoxemia, indicates she has developed ARDS as a complication of pneumonia. These opacities suggest that lung compliance is likely decreased. As a result, more pressure will be needed to inflate her lungs to the desired tidal volume than would be necessary to achieve the same volume in a person with normal lungs. Despite breathing an inspired oxygen fraction of 1.0, her arterial P_{O_2} remains very low. In such cases, it is appropriate to raise the PEEP above 5 cm H_2O. This will increase end-expiratory lung volume and prevent atelectasis and, as a result, improve gas exchange. While the patient's blood pressure may have decreased due to worsening of septic shock related to the pneumonia, it may also be related to initiation of mechanical ventilation. Positive-pressure ventilation increases intrathoracic pressure, which can decrease venous return and cardiac output, particularly when patients are intravascularly volume depleted, as is often the case in sepsis.

INDEX

Note: Page numbers followed by "*f*" indicate figures and those followed by "*t*" indicate tables.

CCS0321